HEAL!

WHOLEISTIC PRACTICES
TO HELP **CLEAR YOUR TRAUMA**,
HEAL YOURSELF,
AND **LIVE YOUR BEST LIFE**

PRAISE FOR HEAL!

Wow. It captivated me. It was an awesome read.
Love the honesty.
The book spoke to me in so many levels;
and finds me understanding what my own journey has been.
I had to get to nature to survive the past several years.
The organics. Good nutrition. Love one another.
A great, great read!

-**JEFF BRAGG**, Chief Nurturer of SuperFood Consulting
(www.superfoodconsulting.com)

HEAL! provides the manual
for accessing the answers to healing you seek!
I REALLY love this book! It establishes a holistic,
lifestyle approach – as clearly this is the way to achieve
wellness and balance... everything is part of a system.
HEAL! provides a blueprint for bringing you to
wholeness and regaining sovereignty over your
physical, mental, and spiritual self.
If you're looking for answers, those answers are
within you, and HEAL! provides the manual for accessing
those answers, tapping into your inner healer, and living
your best life authentically, and with Purpose.

-**GUY BORGFORD**, avid student of consciousness
and owner of Casa de Flujo

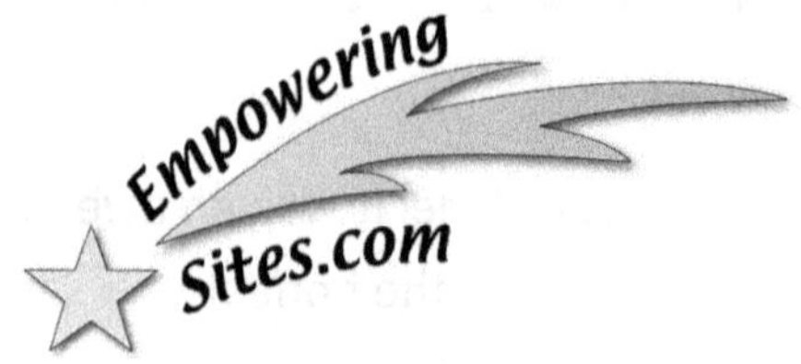

EmpoweringSites.com

To request permissions,
contact the publisher at ceo@empoweringsites.com

Ebook: 979-8-9872520-3-1
Paperback: 979-8-9872520-2-4

Library of Congress Control Number: 2023911724

Edited by Jenny Hansen
Designed by Michelle Fairbanks

This book has been written for informational and educational purposes only. It is not intended to serve as medical advice, a substitute thereof, or a guarantee of outcome and should not be construed as such. It is always recommended to consult your healthcare provider for guidance on any aspect of medical treatment and care. Any use of the information in this book is based on the reader's judgment and is the reader's sole responsibility.

HEAL!

WHOLEISTIC PRACTICES
TO HELP **CLEAR YOUR TRAUMA**,
HEAL YOURSELF,
AND **LIVE YOUR BEST LIFE**

How to heal and become the...
TRUE YOU!

DR. RANDALL S.
HANSEN, PH.D.

DEDICATION

This book is dedicated to everyone who is considering or is on a healing journey.

To become whole again — to be our true selves — we need to have the strength, courage, and dedication to HEAL. Healing takes work, but my hope is that this book becomes a key tool for your *wholeistic* — yes, WHOLE-istic, because true healing makes you whole again — healing journey!

TABLE OF CONTENTS

The Six Wholeistic Elements of Healing

PART THREE: HEALING JOURNEY STORIES

PART FOUR: HEALING QUICK SHEETS

PART FIVE: CONCLUSION & RESOURCES

AUTHOR'S NOTE

How are you? I mean it. How are you doing today? How do you feel about yourself and your life? Are you ready for a healing journey? So really... how are you?

In the words of the great rock band R.E.M., "everybody hurts... sometimes."

This book is written for those of you who are hurting. It's also for those of you who have a brother or sister or spouse or child or parent or best friend who is hurting.

We are more than hurting, though, right? And it's more than sometimes too, right? Who wants to live life through a prism of pain, bitterness, disappointment, rage, guilt, hurt, anger, or shame? Or worse, who wants to feel like they are faking their way through life, feeling numb, resentful, and discouraged?

Why wouldn't you feel angry, depressed, hurt if you were not living your true and authentic life?

We carry negative self-judgments. These are toxic and trapped emotions and beliefs that are simply not true, and yet we cannot seem to shake them. We continually compare ourselves to others, usually not on the winning side of it. We carry guilt and shame, some residual from childhood and earlier parts of our lives. We carry a heaviness with us that has nothing to do with physical weight.

Many of us are lost, disconnected, and searching for something we can't even identify... **searching for our true selves, our true identities... the person we were *meant* to be!**

The world is in crisis — and we need healing. We carry too much pain from past trauma with us — and we carry that trauma in our minds *and* our bodies *and* our souls, which leads to both mental and physical health issues — and more pain. (Some experts refer to this situation as being unregulated, disconnected, or out of balance.)

We are the unhealthiest we have EVER been. We are hurting physically, mentally, and spiritually.

We deserve to be happy, to be loved. We deserve a life filled with joy, right?? We do not have to live with the labels given to us by the medical profession, where everything today seems to be a "disorder." Depression, anxiety, OCD, PTSD, eating disorders, addictions are just *labels that only describe symptoms. These labels have nothing to do with true healing.*

This book takes a ***whole***istic and holistic approach to healing — which means that to truly heal and live your true and authentic life, you need to heal your mind, body, and soul. It is NOT just about mental health... it's about you, it's about your HEALTH because it's all interconnected: your thoughts, your feelings, your emotions, and your beliefs all communicate with your brain, gut, and body — and to be truly HEALED, we need them all to be in alignment.

The work you do with this book — even simply reading it — may trigger some uncomfortable moments and perhaps a few challenges. I ask simply that you stick with it because when you're done, and when you implement your healing protocol, you will begin a journey to the other side of the mountain — the one with the sun and green pastures, singing birds, and beautiful vistas.

This book is not meant to be read in one sitting. My hope is that you will spend some time on each of the six healing techniques in this book, finding the best combination that works for you.

Finally, healing is not a race. Please, take your time. Be patient with yourself and the process. True healing takes time, commitment, and work.

The best place to start your healing journey is simply with one small step: the intention to heal.

You already have all the tools you need to heal. You simply need to begin that healing journey and find the methods that best help you clear that unprocessed trauma.

One final note about triggers in relation to your unresolved trauma. I strongly urge you to lean into those triggers, which will help with discovering the trauma behind the triggers, and then heal from that trauma. We need to stop hiding from our trauma and face it head on so we can heal it.

Can you find healing? My hope is you will find inspiration and motivation from the healing stories in this book.

Finally, who am I to be leading this charge about healing? I have been an educator my entire life and have been in the wellness field for more than two decades. I have seen the hurt and outcomes from trauma. I have also witnessed the lies of marketers and governmental agencies — lies about ingredients, lies about treatments, lies about non-Western healing remedies/modalities.

My purpose in life is educating people about healing — and this book and healing project are my platforms for getting to the truth about trauma and about healing. My goal is to share that knowledge with you so you can take a positive and active role in your healing and in finding your true self.

Along with my educator hat, I am a pragmatist. I seek concrete solutions, not ideals and dreams — nor lies. Traditional pharmacology is not going to heal you. But the methods in this book *will* give you ALL the tools you need to succeed in your TRUE healing journey.

People have asked about my personal healing journey, and I am including a short version of it in the section with the other healing stories. Again... my goal with all these stories is to motivate you to begin or restart YOUR healing journey.

Finally, my daily mantra: "I am happy. I am healing. I am healthy." I share it with you to encourage you to develop something similar for your healing journey.

Know that I am rooting for you! Let's HEAL!

Thank you for reading this book and helping me plant some healing seeds AND spread my message of healing!

*– Dr. Randall "HealingSeed.World" Hansen**

**Curious? Go to HealingSeed.World*

INTRODUCTION

How to Transform Your Life and Live With Truth, Joy, Peace, Fulfillment

More than 140 million babies are born annually into a world with a population of some 8 billion people. In theory, those babies are born into loving homes with parents who know how to properly love and raise their children.

Yet we know that's not the case. Children are left abandoned (even if just for short periods), children are abused/molested, children are exposed to poor living conditions and a lack of proper nutrition. We know the mental health of our children is at its worst ever. We also know childhood obesity is escalating rapidly, as are all sorts of other health conditions.

It's not just children, but young adults as well. According to a recent study of approximately 13,000 people ages 20 to 44 years old, diabetes and obesity — two risk factors for heart disease — are on the rise among this group.

We also know from the research that one in five people were sexually molested as a child and one in four had abusive parents who beat them. About one in four of us were bullied in school. Many "loving" couples engage in verbal and physical violence, which is often witnessed by the children.

So many children experience some sort of trauma — and regardless of what people say about children "having resilience" and "being able to bounce back from tragedy," there's no question that trauma will change everyone it impacts, most especially children. Some experts say almost two-thirds of people experienced significant neglect or abuse as children.

Guess what? You were once a child — it's possible you experienced trauma you can't even recall. The child brain, especially, does a great job of compartmentalizing what it can't really explain, but it also makes incorrect associations — which is why we sometimes have complete meltdowns and outbursts about seemingly trivial things, such as the music playing in the background or the smell of a certain cologne. (We call these things "triggers.")

Still, trauma is not all in childhood. Surgeries, assaults, pandemics, social isolation, poverty, racism, gender discrimination, disabilities, bad/abusive relationships, and chronic pain are ALL traumatic. Being the caregiver for someone — especially someone you love — can be traumatic.

These untreated traumas can poison us in our adult life, greatly affecting our well-being — often leading to depression, anxiety, panic attacks, substance abuse and addiction, stress eating, agitation, confusion, numbness, and dissociation. *Unaddressed trauma can also lead to acting out, putting ourselves in dangerous situations.*

We may think we have put our trauma "in the past," but all trauma leaves traces within us — regardless of how well we think we have dealt with the issues. *Unaddressed trauma can actually change the structure of our brains.*

Problems created by trauma are not limited to mental health issues. Partly because the brain and gut share a strong connection through the brain-gut axis, trauma can also impact physical health, including disrupting our digestion. (And what goes wrong in our gut will cause more issues with our brain — and the cycle between the two continues until the trauma is resolved.)

More recently, many doctors refer to the gut as the second heart. Technically, it's called the enteric nervous system (ENS), which contains two thin layers of more than 100 million nerve cells lining the gastrointestinal tract from the esophagus to the rectum.

Interestingly, the GI tract (gut) produces 95 percent of the body's serotonin — a multifaceted neurotransmitter that helps modulate mood, cognition, reward, learning, memory, and numerous physiological processes. (Historically it was believed that serotonin was only or mainly in the brain.)

Past trauma — of all types — stays with us. It is stored as compressed survival energy, until we can find a way of truly clearing it, not simply masking the symptoms. Untreated trauma leads to a myriad of health and emotional issues, at times robbing us of joy, love, and intimacy, as well as affecting our immune systems.

Even faced with this knowledge, many doctors still take a narrow view on health and actually dismiss the idea that a patient could be experiencing trauma-based physical symptoms, such as gut issues. Ever have someone tell you your symptoms are "psychosomatic" ... that all your health concerns are "in your head?" Have you been blamed or belittled (as many have) for expressing your struggles?

On a side note, we are just beginning to develop an understanding of neuroplastic pain — pain not caused from structural issues, but due to psychophysiological processes that have caused the brain to expect pain and identify pain when there is absolutely no physical pain; it literally is in our heads, as the brain is capable of generating any physical sensation: pain in your neck, pain in your back, nerve pain, muscle pain, toothaches, numbness, burning. In fact, most experts suggest that ***most chronic pain is neuroplastic*** — and it needs to be healed through these same processes of healing your trauma.

Unresolved trauma can have many outcomes. Have you witnessed some of these mini explosions and unhealthy reactions of untended trauma?

- Unexpected, extreme emotional outbursts
- Feelings of anger, fear, unease, sadness
- Strong irritability, hostility
- Nightmares, or, worse, daymares
- Overreaction to a common issue
- Flashbacks
- Difficulty with trusting others
- Paranoia, intense fears

Think I am exaggerating about the degree of trauma in the world? I wish I was. And whether you believe these facts or not, I am glad you are still here — because we all need to heal. We — the collective we of the world — need healing. Having one or more traumas affects how we live, how we love, and the quality of our lives.

Sadly, the most common way to "treat" trauma is by addressing only the symptoms, typically through the use of antidepressants and anxiolytics. Over the last two decades, we have seen a massive increase in the long-term use of these medications in the United States.

Worldwide, the global antidepressant market was valued at $15.6 billion in 2020. This number is expected to escalate to $21 billion by 2030. In the U.S., about 1 in 5 people are on at least one antidepressant medication. Antidepressants are the second most prescribed drugs after antihypertensives (blood pressure medications) — which clearly shows that unresolved trauma affects both the mind and the body .

Other therapies attempt to get to the root of the trauma, but even these therapies have their flaws — especially getting to the root cause(s) of the trauma. The only way to clear all these negative consequences from trauma is to identify it, understand it, and put it properly into your past.

Furthermore, three-quarters of us are self-medicating and engaging in unhealthy coping habits. A recent study from Myriad Genetics found that 77 percent of Americans report using drugs and alcohol or unhealthy eating or sleeping to cope with mental health issues — and those numbers are increasing. While these coping mechanisms will sometimes help a person feel better in the short-term, there are long-term consequences.

**IT'S TIME FOR A PARADIGM SHIFT IN HEALING.
IT'S TIME FOR *WHOLEISTIC* HEALING.**

To truly heal, we need to understand that past traumas can impact every system within our bodies, and that the ONLY way to heal is to clear that trauma, not simply mask the symptoms. To live our true and authentic lives — lives filled more with hope and love — we need to HEAL.

Living with the trauma is bad enough, but at the same time as we are having this trauma buildup inside us, we are also spending too much time on our screens, not getting enough exercise, eating processed and heavily-sugared foods, and not getting enough sleep. Is it any wonder why we are in such desperate need of healing? Our bodies and brains are stressed and struggling. ***We are in trouble.***

Just this past May, the United States Surgeon General Dr. Vivek Murthy released a new advisory calling attention to the public health crisis of loneliness, isolation, and lack of connection in our country.

Do you feel rushed and pressured all the time? Insecure and unsafe? Lonely and alone? Stress eat or self-medicate? Feel like nothing is beautiful? Not engaged with family or friends? Haunted by some fuzzy (or not so fuzzy) memory of some traumatic event? Feel badly about yourself — your job, your status, your looks? Constantly worrying about a nagging issue/problem? Don't like being alone with yourself? Plagued by unknown/unexplained chronic physical pain? Playing the victim — or being the people pleaser? Feeling stuck (in a bad job, relationship)? A sense of being stuck and unfulfilled?

Sadly, without healing, no one can escape the torture of our psyche's attempt to find fault, raise doubts, question our motivations, challenge our ideas of love and happiness, and be our own harshest critic... and even inflict physical pain.

Hang in there! There is hope!

Healing... true healing is transformative!! The rest of this book is designed to help you find your path to true healing and good health... as well as true love and happiness, living an authentic life!

Please remember: While the trauma was caused by someone

else and was out of your control, you **DO** control how to react and deal with pain, how you deal with forgiveness, and how you move toward with healing.

After healing from trauma, people experience wholeness for the first time! It is a true gift.

Recognize that during this healing process forgiveness is essential — forgiveness of yourself first and foremost, but also forgiveness of those who harmed you — as you won't truly heal until you have forgiven everyone for your trauma, your brokenness.

Some last words of advice before you start your healing journey: go slowly and have patience, practice self-love, and be gentle with yourself. *Healing is a process.* But know that true healing is possible; the proof is in this book.

All you need to do is take that first step — and reading this book is a BIG first step!

This book is divided into five sections:

- **Part One: A New Paradigm For True Healing**
  (Key information about the six healing modalities)
- **Part Two: How to Find True Healers**
  (Fact sheets to help you find the healers/healing you seek)
- **Part Three: Healing Stories**
  (Motivational stories showcasing people's healing journeys)
- **Part Four: Healing Quick Sheets**
  (Easy-to-implement tools/techniques for healing)
- **Part Five: Conclusion & Resources**
  (Summation of healing methods and key healing tools)

Finally, to assist you in your healing, and to break up some of the text, I am including a variety of additional information, tips, advice, and quotes using the following techniques:

Author Insights: Interesting and informative healing tidbits the author wants to highlight.

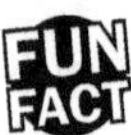

Fun Facts: Nugget-sized bits of fascinating news, data, truths, or history about healing.

Healing Hints: Concise blurbs of expert advice to assist/help with the healing process.

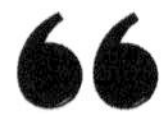

Inspiring Quotes: Short, motivating passages related to healing from a wide range of people.

One final note: I have no agenda here besides seeing you heal. I have no paid program or coaching. I am simply of service in helping the world heal — in helping YOU heal.

Editorial Note: *Some of the work in this book requires changing lifestyles, deep breathing, new foods, and other changes that might put a strain on your body. It is highly recommended that you receive support from a doctor (ideally a naturopath) before jumping into a new healing regimen. None of this work is dangerous for the healthy individual, but it's important to always be safe... especially since our goal is healing and living a joyous and authentic life. And if your current doctor does not support your healing protocol, PLEASE consider finding a new doctor.*

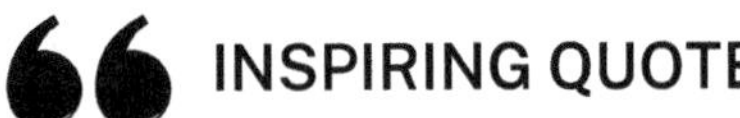

"The doctor of the future will give no medication, but will interest his patients in the care of the human frame, diet and in the cause and prevention of disease." — Thomas A. Edison

PART ONE:

A NEW PARADIGM FOR TRUE HEALING

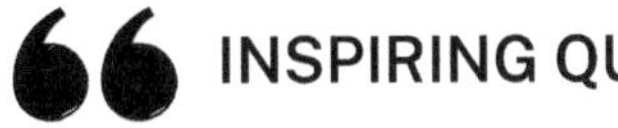

"Forgiveness is not always easy. At times, it feels more painful than the wound we suffered, to forgive the one that inflicted it. And yet, there is no peace without forgiveness." — Marianne Williamson

CHAPTER 1:
What is Trauma... and What We Can Do About It

Let's clear some things up about trauma.

First, trauma is not a disease or condition, but rather a human experience rooted in survival instincts. It is not a brain disorder or a mental problem alone; trauma also impacts our body, our soul. It affects our entire system.

Second, trauma is not what happens TO you, but rather the emotional response to something that we experience, either something horrible that happens to us (directly or indirectly) or when love/safety are withheld. It's what remains in our hearts, our minds, our bodies after the trauma—and those remains are why we can so easily be triggered into an unexpected reaction. Trauma breaks us; our reaction to the trauma is to disconnect from it, thus disconnecting ourselves—from ourself!

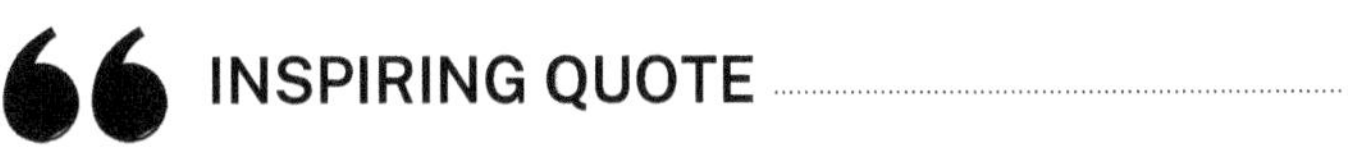

INSPIRING QUOTE

"Trauma is a fact of life. It does not, however, have to be a life sentence." —Peter A. Levine, PhD

Third, it's best to think of trauma as a psychic wound, hurt, defeat that hardens you, typically caused by a single incident or a series of negative events. (Interestingly, trauma is derived from the Greek word for "wound.")

Fourth, just because someone experiences a traumatic event does not mean they will experience trauma.

Fifth, we store/suppress past trauma — the pains from those experiences — deep inside ourselves. We use different words such as "compartmentalizing" or "sweeping under the rug" or "just dealing with emotional baggage" to fool ourselves that we can easily move beyond the trauma... but it's there.

AUTHOR INSIGHT

There has perhaps never been a time before in history when we have experienced a wellness crisis as we are today. Look at all these outcomes from trauma, all on the rise: depression, anxiety, eating disorders, numbing pill prescriptions, addictions, obesity, diabetes, heart disease.

Sixth, childhood trauma is some of the worst, simply because the child's brain does not understand how to process all the information and emotions caused by the event.

Seventh, the result of the trauma often leads to a condition known as post-traumatic stress disorder (PTSD), which is when the trauma memories are so strong they impact your day-to-day functioning. While PTSD is most often discussed in reference to veterans of war, ANYONE who experiences trauma can suffer with post-traumatic stress. (In fact, women are twice as likely to develop PTSD than men.)

Eighth, while trauma is a spectrum of horrible/evil/sad/devastating events ranging from small incidents to major ones, ALL trauma results in emotional and mental baggage that deserves support and healing.

Ninth, while some people are able to fully recover and clear old trauma on their own, many people need assistance in relieving it.

Tenth, trauma can create a negative feedback loop that extends and deepens the trauma reactions, which leads to maladaptive behaviors, and a downward spiral of negative consequences.

HEALING HINT

Trauma represents a profound compression of "survival" energy — energy that has been trapped and needs to be released from the mind, body, and soul.

A LIST OF COMMON CAUSES OF TRAUMA

- Intergenerational (passed-down traumas)
- Abuse (of all forms)
- Assault
- Sexual trauma
- Bullying
- Abandonment/Neglect
- Rejection
- Racism/Colonialism
- War/Combat
- Loss of job
- Financial hardship/loss
- Manipulation
- Terrorism
- Theft/burglary
- Fire/explosions
- Automotive accidents
- Natural disasters
- Medical illnesses/incidents
- Surgery/Medical procedures
- Miscarriage/abortion

- Death/Grief
- Breakup/Divorce
- System-induced separation
- Vicarious trauma
- Witnessing trauma

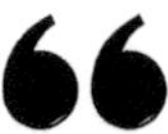

INSPIRING QUOTE

"The greatest damage done by neglect, trauma, or emotional loss is not the immediate pain they inflict, but the long-term distortions they induce in the way a developing child will continue to interpret the world and her situation in it. All too often these ill-conditioned implicit beliefs become self-fulfilling prophecies in our lives. We create meanings from our unconscious interpretation of early events, and then we forge our present experiences from the meaning we've created. Unwittingly, we write the story of our future from narratives based on the past." —Gabor Maté, MD

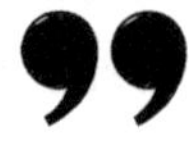

NEGATIVE OUTCOMES RELATED TO TRAUMA

Everyone reacts differently to traumatic events. Some common reactions of people suffering from unresolved trauma:

- Self-medicating
- Addictions
- Eating disorders
- Rage/Hate
- Shame
- Nightmares
- Flashbacks
- Depression
- Paranoia/Anxiety
- Dissociation
- Panic attacks
- Avoidance of all things
- Irrational fears
- Attachment issues
- Fear of abandonment
- Overwhelmed/Mentally paralyzed
- Uncontrollable thoughts (loops
- Easily startled or frightened
- Low self-esteem
- Difficulty sleeping
- Brain fog/trouble focusing
- Overwhelming and chronic guilt/shame
- Uncontrollable anger
- Unwarranted fear
- People-pleasing
- Trying to fix others
- Survivor guilt
- Flight mode overactive
- Falling for a narcissistic partner
- Tolerating abusive behavior
- Toxic perfectionism
- Self-harm (cutting, mutilation)
- Suicidal ideation

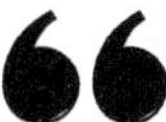

INSPIRING QUOTE

"Trauma binds us to the painful past and makes us continually apprehensive about the future. And trauma may override our intrinsic urge to connect with others, forcing us to fear and avoid those whose care and concern could help and heal us." — James S. Gordon, MD

Furthermore, some of the causes of our suffering and isolation include:

- Living in the past... or the future
- Choosing fear(s)
- Clinging to a (hurt, wrong, false) identity
- Disconnection with the world
- Death (or living with death)
- Being a victim; playing the victim
- Addictions and attachments to things that only bring temporary relief
- Comparison syndrome
- Living a divided life (wearing multiple masks)
- Loss of connection to the Divine

AUTHOR INSIGHT

Until you are completely healed, please recognize and accept that certain people, events, news stories, movies... ANYTHING can reawaken that unhealthy trauma response, often catching us off-guard. We call these things triggers because they are like a speeding bullet to your trauma center — and until you are healed, they will always throw you from calm into the storm.

OTHER OUTCOMES THAT SUGGEST A HEALING JOURNEY

Perhaps you feel trauma is too strong a word for your life experiences — and perhaps you are even questioning the need for a healing journey.

First, no one escapes trauma in one form or another.

Second, your trauma may be expressed in other ways, such as:

- Feeling unfulfilled in your career, with no clear path for finding it;
- You are or have been unsuccessful in all long-term relationships;
- Your life — or parts of it — seems out of balance, out-of-control;
- You struggle with bouts of feeling uninspired, uncreative, and unhappy;
- The same questions keep arising in your mind — for which you have no answers.

METHODS FOR HEALING TRAUMA: A HEALING JOURNEY

No one should have to live with the pain from past trauma, and yet many of us do. Many of us also live with trauma, but are completely unaware of why we feel the way we do.

Many of us have endured a lifetime of smaller traumas, usually ignored/dismissed/compartmentalized experiences, resulting in the equivalent of a lifetime of emotional papercuts — and we know that one or two minor cuts are nothing, but if we have 10 or a hundred, the pain is unbearable.

The key to healing trauma is to get yourself onto a healing journey — ideally one without prescription pills or any other self-medicating with alcohol or other drugs. Sadly, many traumatized people spend their lives self-medicating or being medicated — rather than healing at the core. Prescription drugs have their place, but it's not with healing — where studies reveal the placebo (nonactive medication) has just about the same effects as the meds in MASKING symptoms.

Turn the page to begin discovering the six modalities for healing… and begin your healing journey.

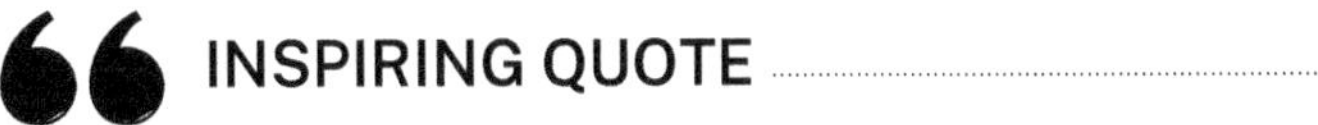

"Love is the healthiest of all emotions. It sustains life at a level of trust, joy, and compassion unrivaled by anything else."
—Deepak Chopra, MD, and Rudolph Tanzi, PhD

HEAL ME WHOLE: UNDERSTANDING TRAUMA CHECKLIST

Here's a quick checklist for Chapter 1 to make sure you gleaned all the important points made about trauma in this chapter.

Remember to actually check off each of these to showcase your understanding!

- ☐ I realize that trauma is NOT a disorder, but rather an experience that impacts my body, my brain, my soul.
- ☐ I understand that trauma-trigger responses come from unprocessed emotions from previous traumatic events.
- ☐ I recognize that because of my upbringing, my family and friends, that the idea of just sweeping trauma under the rug or attempting to "just get over it" are not helpful strategies.
- ☐ I recognize that past trauma may have resulted in me now experiencing post-traumatic stress and that anyone who experiences trauma can have PTSD.
- ☐ I know that I should not be trying to compare my trauma to anyone else's. We all experience trauma as part of life and I need to focus on simply on clearing my trauma so I can live my best life.

CHAPTER 2:
An Introduction to the Six Elements of Healing

If you read the introduction, you know we are in a healing crisis, worldwide. Everyone has been exposed to multiple traumas in their lives, some much more catastrophic than others, but ALL trauma… and with that trauma, all of us have remnants of anger, shame, fear, helplessness, anxiety, depression. Many of us live with some amount of post-traumatic stress and do not even know it. (Numbness is also a trauma reaction.)

How are you doing? If you are not feeling 100 percent, you are not alone! The U.S. Centers for Disease Control and Prevention (CDC) estimates that 50 percent of Americans will be diagnosed with some sort of mental health problem or disorder during their lifetime; worldwide, 280 million people suffer from depression, while 264 million suffer with anxiety disorder. There's no question we are hurting.

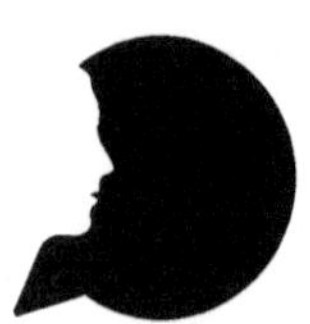

AUTHOR INSIGHT

Healing is a journey, one for which there is no single roadmap that fits all. But with the information in this book, you do have six clear directions to research before choosing one or more of the healing modalities to transform your life for the better.

Have you ever had thoughts like…

- I hate myself;
- I am broken inside;
- I am not living my best life;
- I just do not know what is wrong with me;
- I can't function well on many days;

- Why can't I find my true love? Any love?
- I have unexplainable chronic pain;
- I don't know why I am so hard to love;
- I am tired of battling depression, anxiety;
- I engage in risky behavior to prove I'm alive;
- I wear too many masks to hide my true self;
- I am hurting and just not sure how much more I can take.

I think many of us have been there... and if no one has told you this recently, please repeat this phrase to yourself: ***I deserve a life of meaning and purpose, filled with love, happiness, and good health.***

What stops you from accomplishing living this life, loving this life... is trauma. Researchers suggest that the vast majority of chronic physical, mental, and emotional illnesses are the result of uncleared/unprocessed traumas. You are what you are because of what happened to YOU; there is nothing inherently wrong with you, but you are BROKEN on the inside because of the trauma.

If we are going to live our true, authentic, mission-filled life... we HAVE to HEAL.

The ONLY thing stopping us from true healing is ourselves — and the trauma we have faced/endured.

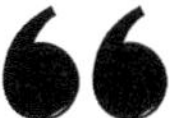 INSPIRING QUOTE

"Experiences of abuse or neglect accumulate in our emotional heart, limiting the flow of love in and out. The toxic residue of incompletely digested mistreatment, disappointment, resentment, or neglect inhibits our ability to give and receive love." — David Simon, MD

When we move from trauma-influenced to healed, we can finally love and accept love (including self-love) — and we know that love is truly transformative, strengthening our overall health, enhancing immune function, boosting digestion, lowering blood pressure, and improving cholesterol levels.

AUTHOR INSIGHT

Sadly, most doctors assume that a physical issue can explain just about all diseases/illnesses — and that the only healing solutions for these are ones that affect the body, such as drugs and surgeries. If your doctor feels this way, please find a new doctor!

At these higher levels of love, the boundaries that separate us seem to dissolve and we focus more on the things that unite us — as true brothers and sisters of humanity.

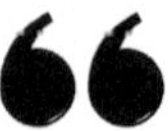

INSPIRING QUOTE

"People with Complex PTSD often have medically unexplained physical symptoms such as abdominal pains, headaches, joint and muscle pain, stomach problems, and elimination problems. These people are sometimes most unfortunately mislabeled as hypochondriacs or as exaggerating their physical problems. But these problems are real, even though they may not be related to a specific physical diagnosis." — Suzette Boon

If you have seen anything I have written in the last year, you know I am on a mission to help everyone find healing. To not only find healing, but to *receive* healing and then to live a true and authentic life. And not only to receive healing and live an authentic life, but to share your healing with others so that they too can receive healing.

I am also a big believer in holistic and *wholeistic* healing — meaning I support natural ways to heal the whole person. I am talking WHOLE-self healing, including the mental, physical, and spiritual — as they are so intrinsically connected that we must address the whole system.... the whole YOU. You cannot have true healing, true health and wellness, true authenticity, without healing your entire whole!

To foster that *wholeistic* healing, I am introducing the ***Healing Wheel: Six Elements of Healing.***

True healing, freeing yourself of old trauma and pain, requires a multidimensional approach — partly because not all therapies work for all people. The key is finding the therapies that resonate with you.

This concept is not new; all we need to do is look at our ancestors in the Indigenous populations of the world, who typically focus on community and healing the whole — not individual parts. These healing experiences included all aspects of the person: physical, mental, spiritual. But it goes deeper than that. The community was a healing community, filled with eating, sharing stories, dancing, singing, loving.

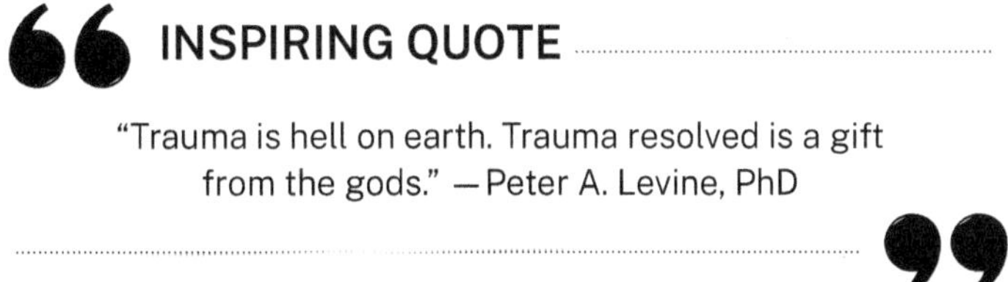

This approach is also similar to the Ayurveda, a medical science that dates back more than 5,000 years, and originated in the southern region of India; it stresses a **holistic** perspective of treating people as **ONE** system — that emotional health is not separate from physical health; that these two systems are one. Ayurveda focuses on healing the physiological, mental, emotional, and spiritual body — the WHOLE system.

Ayurveda translates to the wisdom *(ayur)* of living *(veda)*, and its approach to thriving is aligning one's lifestyle with that of your own individual constitution (or dominant energy), which regulates and sustains every living organism.

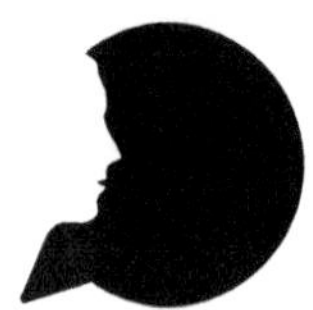

AUTHOR INSIGHT

One of the strongest tools for healing, talk-therapy, is often not available to the people who suffer adversity and trauma; but, a really wonderful alternative is being part of a caring community that supports you and your healing.

Furthermore, this view theorizes that our health depends on our ability to metabolize/use all aspects of life — what we eat, who we interact with, what we watch, our social media activities, the work we do... everything.

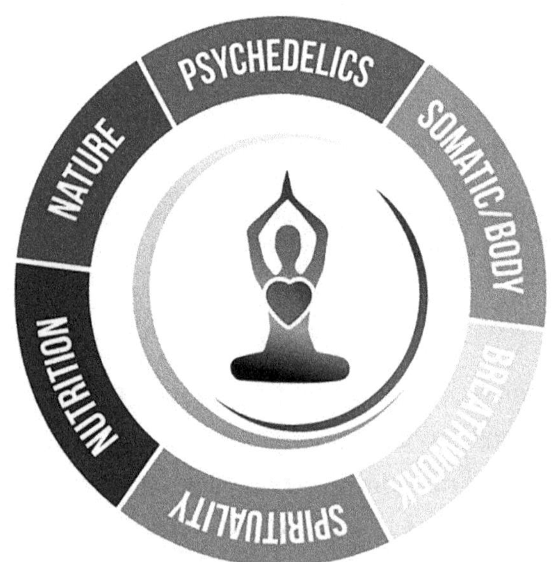

Healing Wheel: Six Elements of Healing

HEALING HINT

Trauma is a highly activated, incomplete biological response to a threat, frozen in time — as reported in a research paper by Payne, Levin, and Crane-Godreau.

The other interesting part of Ayurveda is the vast majority (90%) of its remedies are plant-based, as were most of the Indigenous remedies, which is why so many people in healing focus on the importance and value of plants, alone or in combination — the roots, leaves, fruits, bark, and/or seeds. Included in these plant remedies are cannabis and psychedelic plants, often used alone and/or in combination with other herbs, often in ceremony, for healing within the community.

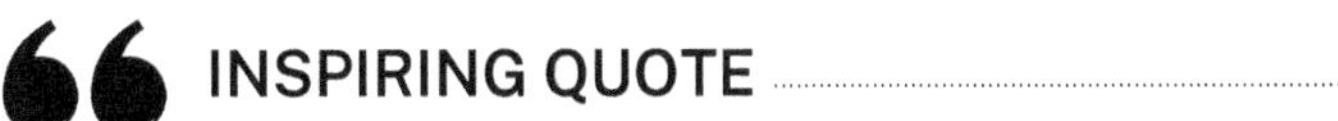

"Ayurveda is a sister philosophy to yoga. It is the science of life or longevity and it teaches about the power and the cycles of nature, as well as the elements." —Christy Turlington

We are all broken, we all have trauma. Many of us struggle with mental wellness. But it's not just about our thoughts and feelings, as many of us also do not eat well, do not spend time in nature, do not exercise consistently. Instead, we suffer or wallow, unsure how to regain control in a world that almost seems to want us sick and hurting.

A world that wants us sick? Sounds a bit sinister, but look at the pharmaceutical industry where mental health treatments simply deal with symptoms, not healing... and we are forced to take those pills daily for the rest of our lives, generating massive profits for the drug companies. Then there's the food industry, often using questionable/cheap sources, chemicals, herbicides, and pesticides in an already-depleted soil.

There's also the government that has banned psychedelics, the least risky drug class in the world, and put them into a classification system that claims they have no medical benefits. And don't get me started on how technology is actually isolating us more than bringing us together in community.

Finally, I am not discounting talk therapy in this model, but in my discussions with people, the talk therapy was generally NOT effective on its own. Furthermore, there is MUCH less talk therapy these days and much more prescribing of antidepressants (for depression; think Zoloft, Lexapro, Celexa) and anxiolytics (for anxiety; think Xanax, Valium) than EVER before. According to one author, most psychiatrists see "drugs as the only treatments worth using."

AUTHOR INSIGHT

A key to healing is believing you can actually and truly heal — and you can when using the principles in this book! Avoid what some refer to as a "nocebo," a negative belief about your healing that can actually increase the likelihood of additional illness.

Over the last two decades, we have seen a massive increase in the long-term use of anxiolytics and antidepressant medications in the United States. Worldwide, the global antidepressant market was valued at $15.6 billion in 2020... and is expected to reach $21 billion by 2030. In the U.S., about 1 in 5 people are on at least one antidepressant medication.

But... WE CAN HEAL... and here's how. The program in this book is designed for you to heal the WHOLE you — body, mind, and spirit — using one or more of these critical healing modalities. To optimize and maintain healing, we must do everything we can for our health... our physical health, mental health, and spiritual health — wholeistic health!

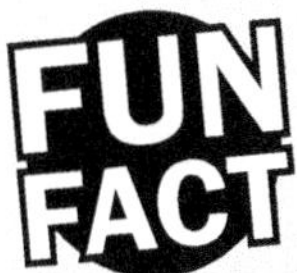

By 1965, there were more than 2,000 published articles involving more than 40,000 patients that noted positive effects with various psychedelics. Much was lost due to the War on Drugs and the scheduling of these medicines as illegal.

THE SIX ELEMENTS OF HEALING

1. Psychedelics. Perhaps the greatest advancement in healing in modern times, though indigenous and native cultures have been using psychedelic plants and fungi for thousands of years. While you may be vaguely aware of psychedelics (and especially LSD) from the War on Drugs and the incredible amount of lies and propaganda, I can assure you these substances are indeed medicines for TRUE healing.

As I discussed in detail in my book, *Triumph Over Trauma,* these psychedelic compounds are being labeled a "breakthrough" medicines, even though they have been around for centuries. In fact, psychedelics were being researched and touted as miracle drugs back in the 1960s — when many therapists used psychedelics as a tool in therapy.

Psychedelic medicines are some of the safest substances on the planet — assuming you do not have serious physical health issues (such as high blood pressure, heart conditions, or serious respiratory issues) or certain mental health conditions (schizophrenia, borderline personality disorder).

We are in the midst a psychedelic renaissance — perhaps even a psychedelic revolution — and it's about time. Research in the field is booming, media interest is reaching a crescendo... and, according to a YouGovAmerica study, one in four Americans say they have tried at least one psychedelic.

Even elite athletes and entertainers are now announcing their use of — and healing with — psychedelics for medicinal, mental health, and other personal reasons. Perhaps the most widely read account is of NFL Quarterback Aaron Rogers, who has stated that Ayahuasca, which he consumed in March 2020 in Peru, has helped increase his "self-love." His story appeared in *Sports Illustrated.*

Other celebrities who have expressed relief and healing from psychedelics include entertainers Joe Rogan, Will Smith (and son Jayden), Susan Sarandon, Rosie Perez, Chelsea Handler, Carrie Fisher, Megan Fox, Reggie Watts, and Seth Rogan; musicians Harry Styles, Kacey Musgraves, Miley Cyrus, Paul Simon, Ben Lee, Sting, and Paul McCartney; NHL's Daniel Carcillo; NBA's Lamar Odom; and boxer Mike Tyson.

Sadly, all psychedelics have been listed as Schedule I controlled substances since the 1970s — the strictest level of control — meaning they are considered to have no current medical use and have a high potential for abuse and/or addiction. This scheduling is absurd, as these substances have proven medical value and have an extremely low potential for abuse/addiction.

Schedule I drugs include LSD, mescaline, MDMA, psilocybin, DMT, Ibogaine, Ayahuasca, and cannabis — but also heroin, quaaludes, and bath salts. Oddly, cocaine, meth, and fentanyl are all Schedule II drugs. Ketamine (perhaps because of its primary use as an anesthetic) is listed as a Schedule III drug.

Interesting to note that two of the most abused drugs — alcohol and tobacco/nicotine — are not even included in this list. (And the absolutely worst "legal" drug still on the market? Sugar.)

Finally, while cannabis is a psychoactive master plant — not a true psychedelic — it is included in this section because people are also finding healing from the medicinal use of this amazing plant.

Learn more about the potential of healing from psychedelics in Chapter 3.

2. Spirituality: Prayer/Meditation/Mindfulness. Without question, "we are spiritual beings — having a human experience," per the powerful words from the French philosopher, Pierre Teilhard de Chardin.

Deep in our hearts, we know there is something more to us, to the world, to the universe than just our physical bodies. (And if you ever have a psychedelic experience, you'll understand this concept even more.)

Spirituality and its related practices can be quite a positive force for healing, especially at a time when so many of us feel disconnected from the people and world around us. More than 3,000 studies indicate that religion and spirituality have a potentially beneficial effect on health, and health is a vital part of healing.

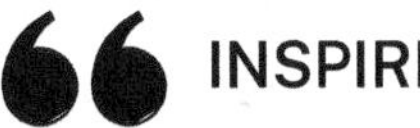

INSPIRING QUOTE

"We can't afford to ignore the potential effect of spirituality and religion on health." — Alexandra Shields, PhD

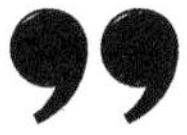

Spirituality is one part of the mind-body-spirit connection, and it may be the most foundational part of who we are. Spirituality is about seeking a meaningful connection with something greater than yourself; it provides a worldview that suggests there is more to life than what we experience on a sensory and physical level.

Spirituality suggests that there is something greater that connects all beings to each other and to the universe itself. And while we have been seeing a decline in organized religious affiliations, we have seen an increase in people identifying as "spiritual but not religious" (SBNR).

Spirituality comes from the Medieval Latin ecclesiastical use of *spiritualis*, "of or pertaining to breathe, breathing, wind, or air; pertaining to spirit, psyche," from *spiritus*, "of breathing, of the spirit."

Spirituality simply means having a connection to something bigger than ourselves (aka, "a higher power"), and it typically involves a search for understanding of our place in the universe. People may describe a spiritual experience as sacred or transcendent... or simply a deep sense of aliveness and interconnectedness. Spirituality practices often result in positive emotions, such as peace, awe, contentment, gratitude, and acceptance.

Finally, spirituality also is about the invisible energy flowing within us; when that energy becomes unbalanced from trauma, illnesses ensue. While some people believe this energy comes from a higher power or deity, others believe it originates from within ourselves, but you should know that everything in the universe consists of energy.

Because the focus is on spirituality — in all its forms — rather than organized religion, it opens us up to numerous avenues for healing, including prayer, meditation, mindfulness. From research, we know these actions can result in reducing our heart rate, lowering blood pressure, decreasing respiration, reducing perspiration, decreasing stress hormones... and increasing anti-aging hormones.

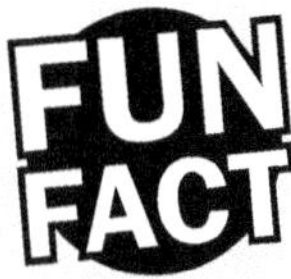

Spirituality can exert a tremendous impact on one's health and promote recovery from trauma and illness, including cancer. Throughout the history of mankind, spirituality and religion have played a major role in healing a variety of physical and mental illnesses. From Torosian & Biddle (2005): "Spirituality and Healing," *Seminars in Oncology.*

One final note, you don't have to be a strongly spiritual person to have a spiritual experience or go on a spiritual journey; to feel the healing energy of nature and the environment. Many of us have experienced a spiritual encounter when standing at the top of a mountain, looking at the night sky, relaxing on the beach, watching the ocean.

According to researchers Matt Snapp and Lisa Hare, there is substantial evidence that spiritual well-being is an important determinant of overall health, longevity, and quality of life.

Learn more about the potential of healing through spiritual practices in Chapter 4.

3. Somatic/Body. There are two key elements within this healing modality — specific body movements to help promote healing and the daily exercise that is important to maintaining good health and to stimulate healing.

Many experts theorize that trauma affects the entire body, not just the mind. Thus, this area of healing operates on the concept that what happens to you in your life is stored not only in your mind, but also in your body—and so you need to clear the trauma from your whole system.

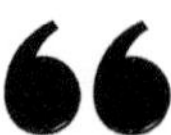

INSPIRING QUOTE

"All emotions, even those that are suppressed and unexpressed, have physical effects. Unexpressed emotions tend to stay in the body like small ticking time bombs — they are illnesses in incubation." —Marilyn Van M. Derbur

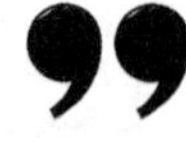

The term somatic comes from the Greek word *soma*, which means "body."

Somatic therapy is a holistic psychotherapeutic that incorporates mind-body exercises and other physical techniques to help people become more self-aware of their bodily reactions, thoughts, and feelings. It uses such techniques to support daily functioning and overall mental healing.

The idea behind somatic therapy is that it helps release the repressed tension/trauma that negatively affects your physical and emotional well-being. Healers use both psychotherapy and physical therapy approaches to help release those built-up tensions that are negatively affecting our physical and emotional well-being.

We also know exercise improves cognition, mood, emotional regulation, and motor function. More specifically, exercise has been shown to foster the release of endorphins, resulting in more positive mental well-being. Finally, in a review of randomized trials of exercise programs, it was found that moderate, aerobic activity three times a week for nine weeks lessened depressive symptoms.

In fact, researchers have discovered regular exercise may be more effective than medication for the treatment of mental illness, as well as improve overall wellness. Published in the *British Journal of Sports Medicine*, the study is one of the most extensive pieces of research to date — and based on their findings, the study concludes that exercise reduced symptoms of depression and anxiety.

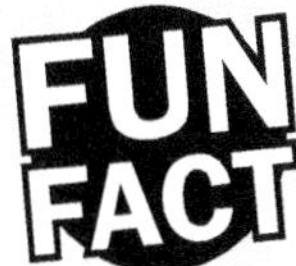

Exercise in all forms induces our whole system to repair itself and keeps us in optimal health. Exercise helps us maintain our physical health and it increases healing.

One final element of this section of healing is body therapy, also a holistic approach — which can include massage and bodywork. Body therapy is based on the belief that sometimes all a person needs to do to improve well-being is to relax, receive, breathe, release... or even play.

Learn more about the potential of healing from exercise and somatic therapy in Chapter 5.

4. Nature. Without question, spending time in nature is healing. In fact, the Japanese have a term for relaxing in nature — shinrin-yoku — which means "forest bathing." It involves opening the senses to the woody aroma of the trees and other plants, the green scenery, and the soothing sounds of streams and waterfalls... because all of these elements play a part in promoting better health and healing.

Simply being in nature induces a state of physiologic relaxation, a true stress-reducer.

Furthermore, a large body of scientific evidence shows that spending time in nature is responsible for many measurable beneficial changes in the body. One of the reasons for these changes are beneficial chemicals produced by trees and plants.

More specifically, recent scientific studies have linked time in nature to symptom relief for many health issues — including heart disease, blood pressure, depression, cancer, anxiety, and attention disorders. Studies also show improvement in cognitive function.

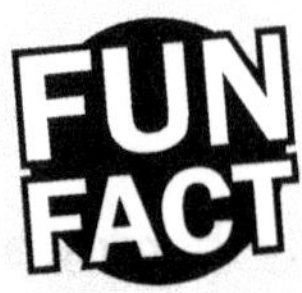

Phytoncides are substances released by trees (and other plants) and generally refers to the aroma of the forest. *Phyton* means "plant" in Latin, and *cide* means to exterminate. Phytoncides play an important role in tree/plant immunity, and are produced to help trees protect themselves from harmful insects and germs.

As a science geek, I feel the most fascinating part of the science is the discovery of phytoncides. The theory is that as people walk in the forest, they inhale phytoncides from the trees, which then increases the number of natural killer (NK) cells within each person. These NK cells are a type of white blood cell that supports the immune system, which is associated with a lower risk of cancer. NK cells are also known for fighting inflammation, which has a role in many major health issues.

Typically, one has to walk/hike to get into the forest, so being in nature can also offer the added benefit of working the body.

AUTHOR INSIGHT

After several traumas started causing my life to spiral out of control, I found so much healing by spending six years in nature, working on restoring the health of a forest (and myself), spending time in nature, working my body and mind, and breathing in the phytoncides.

Learn more about the potential of healing from time spent in nature in Chapter 6.

5. Breathwork. There's transformative power in performing various breathing exercises, including the ability to alter your consciousness for healing. People often perform breathwork to improve mental, physical, and spiritual well-being.

Many people find the idea of breathwork as odd, since breathing is one of those automatic functions (along with our heartbeat and digestion). Breathing is handled by a subconscious part of the brain called the medulla, which automatically controls breathing as well as heart rate and blood pressure.

At its core, breathwork is about taking control of our breathing, and is designed to bring a focus to our breathing, helping to calm our stress levels, lower blood pressure, and bring balance to our bodies.

Breathwork practices have been used by people for thousands of years, and it has roots in yoga. The basic idea of breathwork is to release toxins and stress when you breathe out and nourish your mind and body when you breathe in.

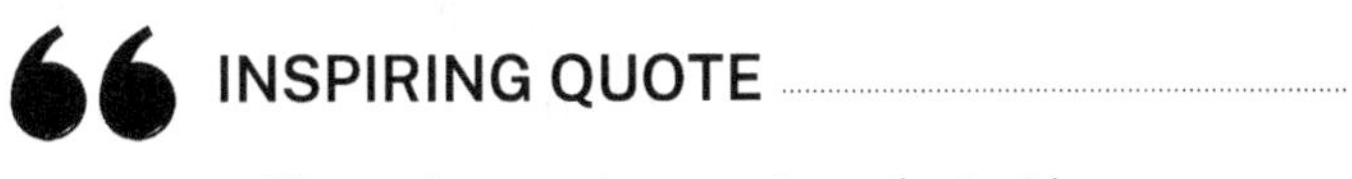

"Some doors only open from the inside.
Breath is a way of accessing that door." — Max Strom

By simply focusing on your breathing, you can help elevate your mood while lowering inflammation levels... all on your way to healing or to help maintain your health and healing.

Two leaders in the "modern" breathwork era include Leonard Orr and Stanislav "Stan" Grof.

Orr, widely considered the *father of conscious connected breath*, discovered the power of breathwork while snorkeling when he experienced memories of his birth. By later experimenting with the technique, he was able to reexamine past traumas and release them from his system. He also experimented with breathwork (via snorkeling) in hot tubs, trying to recreate a feeling of being in the womb and being reborn.

Orr also advocated for the practices of meditation, yoga, cultivating a positive mind, utilizing positive affirmations, eating a healthy diet, and spiritual purification.

Grof is one of the principal developers of transpersonal psychology and the research into the use of non-ordinary states of consciousness for purposes of psychological healing, deep self-exploration, and obtaining growth and insights into the human psyche.

Grof and his wife developed Holotropic breathwork — which was inspired by their work with psychedelics; they were drawn to the transcendental and healing aspects of using consciously-connected breaths (cyclical breathing) for prolonged periods of time.

More recently, Wim Hof and Patrick McKeown have promoted breathing techniques with breath holds to increase physical performance, train athletes, and enter deep meditation.

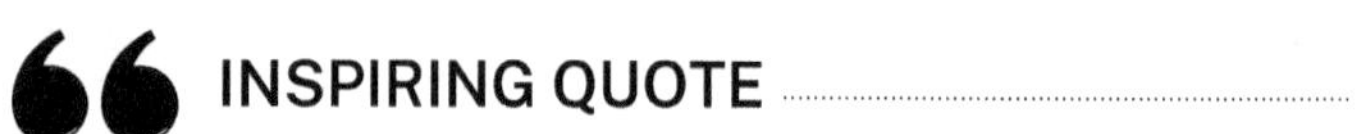

"[With breathwork]... people experience breathing out pain, tension, drama, and trauma into relaxation and peace." — Leonard Orr

Because there are multiple breathwork approaches, the key to success is experimenting and finding the ones that resonate with you and that best works for you.

Learn more about the potential of healing from breathwork in Chapter 7.

6. Nutrition. Whether you believe your body is a temple or simply that we only have one body so we should treat it as best as we can, the result should be the same: a focus on eating healthy, nutrient-dense foods.

Instead, the diets for many of us involve too many meals consisting of low-quality fast-foods or ultra-processed foods from the local grocery store or Walmart. The latest term to describe this "junk" food is hyperpalatable. (Read more here: http://www.empoweringadvice.com/change-grocery-shopping.html)

Many of us are literally eating ourselves to death... it's so bad, we even have an acronym for it, SAD: Standard American Diet, which consists of ultra-processed foods, added sugars and salts, artificial flavors and colorings, refined/bleached grains, as well as *toxic* fats and oils. About 50 percent of the calories in SAD come from simple carbohydrates! Missing from SAD are fresh fruits, vegetables, whole grains, and lean proteins.

We can see multiple indicators of the problems/implications with our food system and the "foods" we consume:

- Obesity (now at the highest levels ever)
- Type 2 diabetes (at epidemic levels)
- Cardiovascular disease
- Coronary artery disease
- Hypertension
- Stroke

- Cancer
- Brain fog/memory issues/dementia
- Kidney/gallbladder disorders
- Osteoarthritis
- Gastroesophageal reflux disease (GERD)

How concerned should we be? The World Obesity Federation's 2023 atlas predicts that 51 percent of the world, or more than 4 billion people, will be obese or overweight within the next 12 years — with the rates of obesity rising quickly among children and in lower income countries.

The solution is going back to the basics — eating whole/real foods... foods that are as close to their natural state as you can find: unprocessed, without a label or a barcode (thus, ideally grown yourself or purchased from a farmer's market). The answers are in the produce and fresh meat sections. Purchase fresh (or frozen) vegetables and fruits, nuts, eggs, fish, and truly pasture-raised poultry and meats. Note that none of these foods have any added fats, sugars, or artificial ingredients.

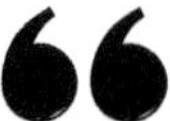

INSPIRING QUOTE

"Today's children are MORE at risk from poor nutrition than they are from drugs, alcohol, and tobacco COMBINED." — Dr. David Katz

We also need to be smarter with our meal planning. Why not cook one or two big meals on the days you're not working and save the leftovers for your busy days? Crockpots and Instant Pots are great tools for preparing meals without too much time spent in the kitchen — and a much better alternative to fast foods.

At the same time, soil health on U.S. farms is the worst it has ever been, as industrial farming has destroyed the soil through raising mono-crops, as well as the use of chemicals, herbicides, and pesticides ... thus, our conventionally-grown fruits and vegetables are not as nutrient-dense as in the past AND contain pesticides. The only real solution is growing your own or only buying from producers raising organically (or at least following organic principles).

HEALING HINT

Simply changing from eating processed foods to cooking from scratch, to removing as much added and excess sugars, and switching to using *beneficial oils* (coconut, avocado, olive) are three small things you can do that will have a MAJOR impact on your health.

Food can truly be our medicine — but we need to be eating the RIGHT foods to make it true.

Learn more about the potential of healing from better nutrition in Chapter 8.

What About Conventional Medicine? Can We Heal Through it? NO.

We have a medical community that seems to do a great job in patching us up to get back out there into our careers and lives... but that has nothing to do with ***true*** healing.

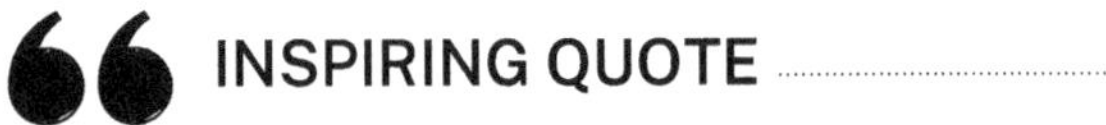

"All of the diagnoses that you deal with–depression, anxiety, ADHD, bipolar illness, post-traumatic stress disorder, even psychosis — are significantly rooted in trauma. They are manifestations of trauma. Therefore the diagnoses don't explain anything. The problem in the medical world is that we diagnose somebody and we think that is the explanation." — Gabor Maté, MD

Please take note: The medical community is much more about relieving your ***symptoms***, NOT addressing the core issues — and certainly NOT about *healing*.

Don't believe me? Look at these scenarios:

- You go to the doctor feeling an overwhelming sadness — and the doctor prescribes an antidepressant, which (in theory) will help mask some of the sadness.
- You go to the doctor feeling anxious and on-edge — and the doctor prescribes you an anxiolytic (such as Xanax, Valium) to help mask the anxiety, to "decrease abnormal excitability."
- You go to the doctor with acid reflux that you can't seem to control — and the doctor prescribes drugs that block acid production — so you can keep eating as you like.
- You go to the doctor for chronic pain — and the doctor prescribes you a pain killer and an anti-inflammatory drug (and maybe even a steroid) so that you can get back to your busy day.
- You go to the doctor struggling with all the changes in your body from perimenopause — and the doctor prescribes you a low-dose antidepressant to help you through the "tough days."

The problem is systemic. The medical community has programmed us into thinking there is (or should be) a pill for every ailment. Who hasn't seen one — or one billion — of the pharmaceutical ads showing us how much more life could be if we only took their drug.

Let's look at few more data points:

- Worldwide, the global antidepressant market is BIG business, valued at $15.6 billion in 2020... and is expected to reach $21 billion by 2030. In the U.S., about 1 in 5 people are on at least one antidepressant medication.
- In terms of all prescription drugs, Americans filled almost **4 billion** prescriptions in 2020 — nearly 13 prescriptions for every man, woman, and child in the United States. According to the U.S. Food & Drug Administration (FDA), nearly *two-thirds of all patient visits to physicians result in one or more prescriptions.*
- Many Americans have also been suffering through the opioid epidemic, moving from OxyContin to heroin to fentanyl. In the last two decades, more than a million people have died from drug overdoses — with the vast majority of those deaths from opioids.
- In the U.S., alcohol consumption and associated deaths are also on the rise; in fact, the U.S. Centers for Disease Control and Prevention (CDC) reports that alcohol-related deaths in the U.S. rose 30% during the years 2020 and 2021.
- Suicide rates are some of the highest they have ever been — especially among veterans and first responders. Suicide is the 12th leading cause of death in the U.S., and in 2020, 45,979 people killed themselves — an average of 130 suicides per day. During that same period, about 12.2 million people seriously thought about suicide and approximately 1.2 million people attempted suicide.

But the problem also rests with us. Yes, we have been programmed into thinking we just need to see our doctor and get a prescription, but many of us also prefer to do the easy work of taking a pill rather than the harder work of doing something to actually address the core problem/trauma.

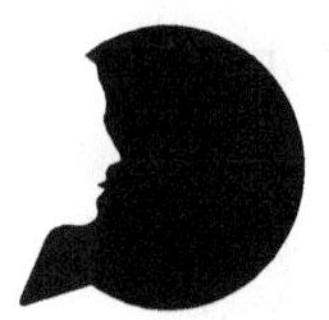

AUTHOR INSIGHT

The first time I knew we had a prescription drug problem — with our doctors prescribing too many — was about 20 years ago. I went for my annual wellness check with my primary care physician (same one I had for years), and the FIRST question out of his mouth was, "do you need any prescriptions?" He had **never** written me a prescription. *Whoa.*

The way to heal, then, is not through medicating (or self-medicating) our pains and ailments, but doing the work that gets us face-to-face with the real issue, the real trauma(s) — so that we can clear them and live a more authentic, happy, and healthy life.

Trauma robs us of our health, robs us from love, robs us from living our authentic lives. We deserve to be healthy. We deserve to be loved. We deserve to live fully as ourselves (and not hiding behind masks).

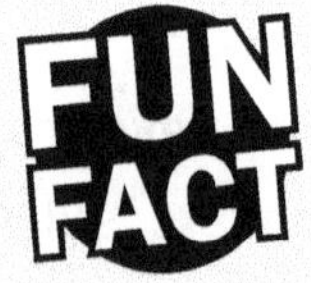

If you look at the meaning behind the word "heal," it means to bring wholeness: heal (v.)
Old English *hælan* "cure; save; make whole, sound and well," from Proto-Germanic *hailjan*, literally "to make whole."

Our conventional model is NOT healing. We are not getting healed. The system is broken. We have to reprogram ourselves from going down the conventional route.

Healing comes from doing the inner work; healing comes from uncovering and clearing past traumas; healing comes from finding a supportive community; healing comes from within —

we just need to find the tools necessary so that we can do that work of healing.

Are you ready for TRUE healing? For discovering your TRUE self? The TRUE you?

What if you could heal completely — physically, mentally, spiritually? What if you could heal and grow into your true and authentic self? The person you were meant to be before you experienced trauma.

Get started with healing — with making yourself whole — by turning the page and learning about the six healing modalities for trauma.

HEAL ME WHOLE: UNDERSTANDING THE SIX ELEMENTS OF HEALING CHECKLIST

Here's a quick checklist for Chapter 2 to make sure you gleaned all the important points made about holistic healing in this chapter.

Remember to actually check off each of these to showcase your understanding!

- ☐ I realize that holistic methods of healing get to the core of the trauma and provide me with the tools to truly heal.
- ☐ I recognize that while psychedelics may not be for everyone, these emerging medicines offer great hope for true healing.
- ☐ I understand the importance of spirituality's impact on my health and am looking forward to going on a spiritual healing journey.

- ☐ I comprehend the importance of removing trauma that has built up in my body, as well as the importance of exercise is to my health.
- ☐ I know that spending time in nature can be quite healing, grounding me to the Earth. I plan to schedule time for enjoying the tranquility and peace of forest bathing.
- ☐ I grasp the transformative power of using breathing techniques and exercises to alter my consciousness, expand my mind, and find healing.
- ☐ I value the importance and role of food and nutrition in healing and health. It's not about fad diets, but of eating nutrient-dense (and ideally organic) whole foods.

CHAPTER 3:
Psychedelics

Psychedelics are a classification of substances that include plants and chemical compounds that produce unique experiences that can result in true healing, getting to the root cause of trauma, and helping the journeyer understand the nature of the trauma and how to recover from it.

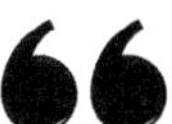

INSPIRING QUOTE

"We're seeing across the United States and beyond a resurgence of plant-based medicine. Whether the plant is cannabis or psilocybin-producing mushrooms, people are finding genuine relief from a variety of ailments from these plants." —Nathan Howard

These substances we refer to as medicines have been used in healing and sacred ceremonies for centuries by Indigenous peoples around the world. Furthermore, many of these medicines were studied in the last century, showing promising results—until the government banned all of them.

Also referred to as entheogens or empathogens, these psychedelic medicines are psychoactive substances that produce alterations in conscious experience. Traditional psychedelics (including LSD, psilocybin, mescaline, and DMT) affect the brain's serotonin system, primarily by binding to the serotonin 2A (5HT-2A) receptor. Other substances with known hallucinogenic properties (such as ketamine, MDMA, and others) have different targets in the brain but still produce some psychedelic effects.

All true psychedelics have been listed as Schedule I controlled substances since the 1970s — the strictest level of control — meaning they are considered to have no current medical use and have a high potential for abuse and/or addiction, both of which are incorrect about psychedelics.

Schedule I drugs include LSD, mescaline, MDMA, psilocybin, DMT, Ibogaine, Ayahuasca, and cannabis — but also heroin, quaaludes, bath salts. Oddly, cocaine, meth, and fentanyl are all Schedule II drugs. Ketamine (perhaps because of its primary use as an anesthetic) is listed as a Schedule III drug.

Interesting to note that two of the most abused drugs — alcohol and tobacco/nicotine — are not even included in this list of "dangerous" substances.

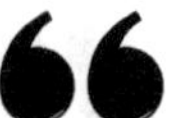

INSPIRING QUOTE

"Psychedelics are illegal not because a loving government is concerned that you may jump out of a third story window. Psychedelics are illegal because they dissolve opinion structures and culturally laid down models of behavior and information processing. They open you up to the possibility that everything you know is wrong." — Terence McKenna

Happily, we are in a grand psychedelic renaissance, and research studies are being conducted globally.

These powerful medicines, demonized by governments all around the world, are continuing to show great promise in contributing to the healing of many mental health issues. While research is ongoing, this is a quick list of the conditions for which early analysis of evidence illustrates psychedelic medicines show great promise as novel and breakthrough therapies:

- Depression: MDMA, psilocybin, LSD, DMT, ketamine, mescaline
- Anxiety: MDMA, psilocybin, LSD, ketamine, mescaline
- Post-traumatic Stress: MDMA, Ayahuasca, ketamine, psilocybin
- Obsessive Compulsive Disorder (OCD): psilocybin, ketamine
- Eating Disorders: MDMA, Ayahuasca, ketamine, psilocybin
- Substance Use Disorder/Addiction: MDMA, ketamine, Ibogaine, LSD, Ayahuasca, mescaline, psilocybin
- Suicidal Ideation: ketamine, mescaline
- Cluster headaches/migraines: LSD, microdosing psilocybin, LSD, DMT
- Attention Deficit Disorder (ADHD): microdosing LSD, psilocybin

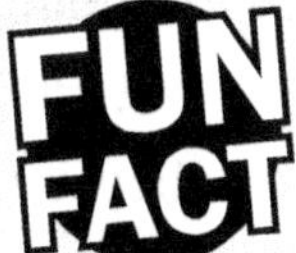

People have been using psychedelic plants and fungi for thousands of years — since time immemorial — for healing, for insights, for religious and spiritual ceremonies, for community.

Beyond the aforementioned therapeutic effects, many participants report lasting benefits from psychedelic medicines, including:

- Improved self-esteem
- Enhanced mood
- Deepened spirituality, divinity
- Greater positivity
- Stronger sense of connectedness
- Heightened optimism
- Enriched world view
- Mindfulness (and a calmer mind)
- Psychological flexibility

Based on anecdotal data, these medicines are some of the fastest ways to get to true healing. Many people report that one psychedelic experience is like 7 years of talk-therapy... and just about everyone who has undergone a psychedelic journey describes it as one of the most profound experiences of their lives.

That said, psychedelics exist in a murky environment these days. Some cities and states in the U.S. have enacted laws to either decriminalize these substances and/or force the rescheduling of some of the substances from Schedule 1 so that they can be used in therapeutic settings. For the vast majority of us in the U.S., all psychedelics are illegal, except for ketamine; but ketamine is not legal in all states and is quite expensive.

Furthermore, consuming psychedelics without completing the integration of your journey into your regular life is like going to an expert for advice and then completely ignoring that advice. One of the biggest misunderstandings of psychedelics is that they are a cure-all... that they are miracle medicines.

Psychedelics are miraculous, but not magical. Psychedelics have proven power to change the brain and help people with numerous mental conditions, but their power comes from being a tool users can employ to heal themselves. **<u>You</u>** are responsible for doing the work!

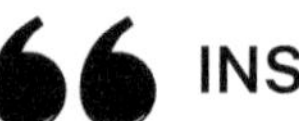

INSPIRING QUOTE

"With psychedelics, if you're fortunate and break through, you understand what is truly of value in life. Material, power, dominance, and territory have no value. People wouldn't fight wars, and the whole system we have currently would fall apart. People would become peaceful, loving citizens, not robots marching around in the dark with all their lights off." —Gary Fisher

Psychedelics open certain portals and increase awareness and knowledge of hidden and suppressed events/traumas — but participants MUST complete the work of integrating the psychedelic experiences into real change in their lives. Your goal is to make sense of the lessons and messages you received during your journey and determine how they can be applied to your everyday life.

To attempt to obtain healing from these medicines, you are currently faced with four choices:

- Join a clinical trial (https://psychedelic.support/resources/how-to-join-psychedelic-clinical-trial/)
- Go abroad to one of many legal retreats, including Europe, Mexico, and South America (https://retreat.guru/)
- Find a qualified psychedelic-assisted therapist
- Hire a professional guide or tripsitter
- Attend an underground healing center ceremony (but only after carefully vetting)
- Source the medicine yourself, or from the underground marketplace

HEALING HINT

If you are having trouble with journaling or integrating your psychedelic experience, you may want to hire an integration coach, who can guide you in understanding your journey and how to implement into your life. Search on your own, connect with a psychedelic society in your area, or find a coach from MAPS (https://integration.maps.org/).

Your two options with the intentional use of psychedelics: macrodosing and microdosing:

- Macrodosing: Consuming a large enough dose of a psychedelic medicine to have a hallucinogenic experience — the typically profound, classic psychedelic journey. A macrodose tends to result in drastic perceptual, cognitive, and emotional changes. A macrodose could be anywhere between a threshold dose — the dose at which perceptual changes just become noticeable — and a heroic dose, where one often has deep and intense effects — such as ego death/dissolution.
- Microdosing: consuming a tiny fraction (5-10 percent) of a full dose of a psychedelic medicine, allowing many of the benefits of the medicine to be utilized without the hallucinogenic (psychedelic) experience. While research has been mostly anecdotal, we are seeing studies that suggest that microdosing can bring about some of the benefits observed with full-dose treatment without causing the intense and sometimes negative hallucinatory experiences. For others, microdosing is also used as a tool for gently "getting to know" a psychedelic medicine before deciding to complete a macrodose journey.

The science behind why psychedelics seem to have such profound effects on the brain comes down to neuroplasticity — what allows neural networks in your brain to change through growth and reorganization — in response to life experiences — creating new neurons and building new networks.

Emerging research suggests that there's a clear link between psychedelics and neuroplasticity, and that using psychedelics may help you make long-term, positive changes to your brain. Your brain actually has increased neural plasticity when consuming psychedelics, providing an opportunity to make significant changes to your life that may last a long time.

These psychedelic medicines are:

- Consciousness-expanding
- Perception-changing
- Mind-manifesting
- Brain network-rearranging
- Mystical/spirituality-enhancing
- Love/bliss-boosting
- Life-enriching

AUTHOR INSIGHT

I am not a psychonaut by any stretch of the imagination, but I have now journeyed on several of these medicines, including Ayahuasca, MDMA, psilocybin, and LSD. Of those four, there is absolutely no question, my medicine is LSD. The entire concept and outline for my last book, *Triumph Over Trauma*, came through a "digital download" from the medicine.

THE MAJOR PSYCHEDELIC MEDICINES

Each psychedelic medicine has its own unique attributes and effects, so it's important to do your research and discover the best medicine for you.

Psilocybin/Magic Mushrooms: More formally known as psilocybin to get away from the recreational use stigma of "magic mushrooms," fungi with psychoactive properties have been used for as many as 10,000 years — maybe even longer. Since the 1950s, psilocybin has been used extensively in clinical research, with more than 40,000 patients receiving this medicine without serious adverse events. Psilocybin is probably the most widely used psychedelic because of its widespread availability and its deep, inward journeys.

Ayahuasca: A plant-medicine brew known as the "vine of the soul" is prepared from the combination of the Ayahuasca vine and the leaves of the Chacruna shrub that grows naturally in the Amazon in South America. This DMT-infused "tea" has been used for healing and community for thousands of years. While Ayahuasca can be found in underground centers in the United States and in limited religious centers, most people still travel to Peru (or Mexico or Costa Rica), where it is legal.

Mescaline: This psychedelic medicine is found in just a handful of cacti and its use can be traced back 6,000 years, to prehistoric peoples participating in ceremonies in the Rio Grande area of Texas. It also has a long history of use by Indigenous peoples in Central and South America. The two cacti with the highest amounts of mescaline are the San Pedro (also known as *Huachuma*) and peyote cacti, though it is also found in the Peruvian torch, the Bolivian torch, and to an even lesser amount in other species of cacti.

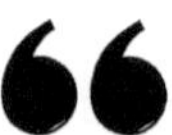

INSPIRING QUOTE

"LSD is a psychedelic drug which occasionally causes psychotic behavior in people who have NOT taken it." —Timothy Leary, PhD

LSD: Swiss chemist Albert Hoffman first derived LSD in 1938 from a chemical (lysergic acid) derived from ergot, a fungus that infects grain. LSD-assisted psychotherapy was used in the 1950s and early 1960s by psychiatrists, with very positive results for thousands of patients—and accepted as a mainstream therapy tool. During this same period, six international conferences, more than 1,000 scientific papers, and several books were written about the use of LSD in psychiatry.

MDMA: First developed by scientists at Merck in 1912 when they were looking for a parent compound to synthesize medications that control bleeding. Like LSD, MDMA was used by some psychiatrists in therapy during the late 1970s and early 1980s — despite that the drug had never undergone any clinical trials nor been approved for human use by the FDA. Psychiatrists found that MDMA was a useful tool in helping patients open up for talk therapy.

AUTHOR INSIGHT

My colleague Matt Zemon likes to say that while psychedelics are for everyone, not everyone should take psychedelics — and I agree. Psychedelic medicines are showing phenomenal results in scientific studies and anecdotal stories of healing, but not everyone is cut out for a deep psychedelic experience, whether for health or personal reasons. That said, one option for obtaining some of the benefits of psychedelics without the hallucinations is through microdosing these medicines.

Ketamine: A more recent discovery and the only "legal" psychedelic, ketamine dates back to 1962 when it was first synthesized by American scientist Calvin Stevens at the Parke Davis Laboratories; it's a medication primarily used for induction and maintenance of anesthesia. It induces dissociative anesthesia, a trance-like state providing pain relief, sedation, and amnesia — and is considered a hallucinogen — but not a classic psychedelic (such as LSD, psilocybin, mescaline, DMT). As a dissociative, ketamine can make people feel disconnected from their physical bodies.

Ibogaine: A naturally-occurring psychoactive substance with dissociative properties found in the roots of shrubs in the family

Apocynaceae such as Tabernanthe iboga, and native to the rain forest of Central and West Africa. Ibogaine is used by Indigenous peoples in low doses to combat fatigue, hunger, and thirst, and in higher doses, as a sacrament in religious rituals. Ibogaine has been used for centuries by African Indigenous people, and was first observed/reported by French and Belgian explorers in the 19th century.

DMT: Is found naturally-occurring in many plants, animals — **and even people** — and has been used (indirectly) by Indigenous people are centuries. (DMT has been found in 400 kinds of plants and fungi.) The largest percentage of the plants that contain DMT are native to South America. DMT is also referred to as the "spirit molecule" due to the intense psychedelic experience it offers and that most people report seeing God, the Creator, and otherworldly creatures.

HEALING HINT

If you decide to try one of these psychedelic medicines, you MUST be willing to do the work after the experience. The medicine will interact with you and show you what is wrong; the trauma you experienced but had forgotten, what needs to be fixed, even how to fix these things, but the medicine — the psychedelic experience — is just the beginning of a long journey of healing and work on changing your life. We call this "after" process integration, and it will be covered in detail later in the book — because it is something you need to do with any of these healing modalities.

CANNABIS: NOT A PSYCHEDELIC, BUT A MASTER HEALING PLANT

Cannabis is a master plant that is worthy of study and medicinal use — one that can even have some psychoactive properties — though most experts do not consider cannabis to be a psychedelic. Still, it's a healing plant that has been used medicinally for centuries — and needs to be included in the discussion of healing plants.

Cannabis (and the cannabinoids within it) is being touted as a miracle drug and a natural cure for many conditions and ailments, but please conduct your own investigation before diving into this plant medicine.

That said, research is discovering amazing benefits from cannabis, especially in relation to post-traumatic stress, inflammation, anxiety, pain, and sleep. (Other names associated with cannabis include hemp, CBD, marijuana, THC.)

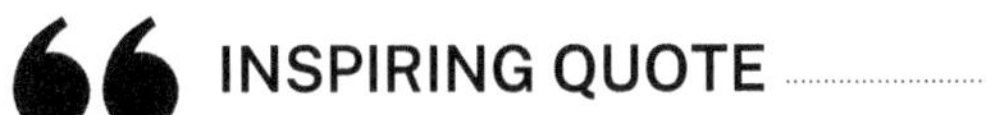

"Cannabinoids are now known to have the capacity for neuromodulation, via direct, receptor-based mechanisms, at numerous levels within the nervous system. These provide therapeutic properties that may be applicable to the treatment of neurological disorders, including anti-oxidative, neuroprotective effects, analgesia, anti-inflammatory actions, immunomodulation, modulation of glial cells and tumor growth regulation. Beyond that, the cannabinoids have also been shown to be remarkably safe with no potential for overdose." — Gregory T. Carter, MD

Cannabis is the name used for two varieties of the *Cannabis Sativa* plant; hemp plants (that contain less than .3 percent THC) and cannabis plants that contain higher (pun intended) amounts of THC (and less CBD), are often referred to as incorrectly as marijuana.

AUTHOR INSIGHT

I have used multiple CBD products created from hemp to help deal with nightly pains and sleep disturbances. For me, the CBD is magical; it puts me in a relaxed state before bed, reduces my pains to zero, and helps me get a full night of sleep. I have also found my demeanor and outlook during the day as better, brighter — and less fear of a poor night's rest.

CBD — or cannabidiol — is one of more than 540 phytochemicals found in cannabis, and researchers are continuing to find new versions of the CBD that provide a multitude of benefits. THC (delta-9-tetrahydrocannabinol) is the element that produces a "high." (Interestingly, there are more than 100 known cannabinoids found in the cannabis plant — and each offers potential health benefits.)

Current medicinal research results with cannabis:

- **Pain and Inflammation Reduction.** CBD has been proven to help reduce inflammation and the neuropathic pain it can cause. Clinical studies have confirmed that CBD reduces the levels of pro-inflammatory cytokines and inhibits T-cell proliferation.
- **Addiction Management.** CBD has been found useful in helping people who suffer from drug and alcohol addiction by reducing cravings and anxiety in recovering patients.
- **Depression and Anxiety.** CBD has been shown to be effective in treating generalized anxiety disorder, panic disorder, social anxiety disorder, obsessive-compulsive disorder, and post-traumatic stress.
- **Calmness of Mind and Deeper Sleep.** CBD helps calm the mind and moves it into a rest and digest state. A calm mind leads to a deeper sleep — which has many of its own health benefits.

- **Neuroprotection.** Several studies suggest cannabis can help protect people from neurodegenerative diseases, including Alzheimer's, ALS, Huntington's, Multiple Sclerosis (MS), and Parkinson's.
- **Soothing Chemotherapy's Negative Side Effects:** Cannabis has been shown to help relieve nausea and other negative side effects in cancer patients taking chemotherapy.
- **Other promising benefits of CBD.** Researchers are studying the anti-seizure and anti-cancer properties of cannabis — as well as its potential to help with GI disorders (such as irritable bowel syndrome (IBS), inflammatory bowel disease (IBD), Crohn's, and ulcerative colitis). There's also growing evidence that cannabinoids can help fight certain types of cancers. Additionally, there is evidence that cannabis has a direct impact on regulating insulin and blood sugar, which can have an impact on weight loss and diabetes.

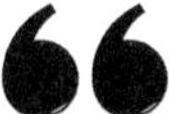

INSPIRING QUOTE

"I have seen many patients with chronic pain, muscle spasms, nausea, anorexia, and other unpleasant symptoms obtain significant — often remarkable — relief from cannabis medicines, well beyond what had been provided by traditional (usually opiate-based) pain relievers." — David Hadorn, MD, PhD

To learn more about these psychedelic medicines, I encourage you to review some of the free resources available on the *Triumph Over Trauma* website; even better, for full details, buy a copy of the book! (When you buy the book, you help yourself find healing AND help others heal because all the proceeds are going to nonprofits in the psychedelic healing space.) Website: https://triumphovertraumabook.com/

HEAL ME WHOLE: UNDERSTANDING THE HEALING FROM PSYCHEDELICS CHECKLIST

Here's a quick checklist for Chapter 3 to make sure you gleaned all the important points made about healing via psychedelic medicines in this chapter.

Remember to actually check off each of these to showcase your understanding!

- ☐ I realize that psychedelic medicines offer much hope for true healing.
- ☐ I understand the two main methods for using psychedelics for healing — macrodosing for a full-on psychedelic experience and microdosing for healing without the hallucinogenic effects.
- ☐ I recognize the importance of understanding and finding the best psychedelic medicine for my healing journey.
- ☐ I comprehend there are multiple methods for obtaining healing via psychedelics, including clinical trials, legal retreats, psychedelic guides and coaches, and underground sources.
- ☐ I grasp the science behind psychedelics, including the concept of neuroplasticity, and that psychedelics have long-term, positive effects on the brain.
- ☐ I now understand that we have been lied to for decades about the so-called dangers of these substances, while also understanding that many plant medicines have been used safely for thousands of years.
- ☐ I know that while cannabis is not a psychedelic, it is truly a healing master plant that should be investigated and possibly used for my healing journey.

CHAPTER 4:
Spirituality, Including Prayer/ Meditation/Mindfulness

Research has shown the value of quieting the mind through relaxed reflection — reducing stress, lowering blood pressure, improving mood and cognitive function, calming the body, and slowing down the aging process. (These results can come from as little as 15 minutes per day in quiet reflection.)

We are spiritual creatures, no question. But spiritual does not necessarily mean religious; it means that more people believe in some sort of higher power, some Divine power, but not necessarily in some organized religious order.

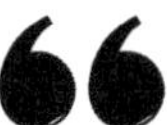

INSPIRING QUOTE

"Spiritual healing occurs as we begin to consciously reconnect with our essential being — the wise, loving, powerful, creative entity that we are at our core." — Shakti Gawain

There are many elements of spirituality: the belief in things greater than us, the appreciation of beautiful moments, the quieting of the brain, a sense of connectedness with others/the world, and compassion/empathy/love for our fellow humans of the world.

That said, it's clear that for many of us, we have lost our connection to the Divine — whether we call that the Universe, God, Jesus, Jehovah, Almighty, Creator, Bhagavan, Buddha, or Allah.

AUTHOR INSIGHT

I was sexually assaulted by an Episcopal priest, and we know quite well that these abuses happen across many religious organizations — Catholic, Protestant, Christian, Hindu, Islam. Some of our greatest traumas occur in sacred places and spaces, which is yet another reason people are leaving organized religions for their own personal relationships with the Divine.

Spiritual healing is the practice (and experience) of trying to rebuild that connection — about restoring, harmonizing, and balancing our spirit/soul. For those who never had much of a spiritual life, spiritual healing can lead to a great spiritual awakening.

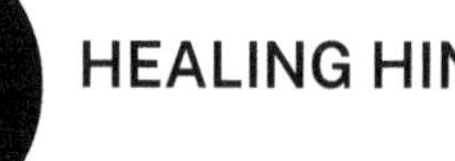

HEALING HINT

Many people around the world credit personal healings, as well as positive changes to the world around them, to prayer.

Spiritual healing can come from a variety of practices:

- Prayer
- Meditation
- Mindfulness
- Affirmations
- Inner child work
- Shadow work
- Solitude and introspection
- Spending time in nature
- Self-love and self-care practices

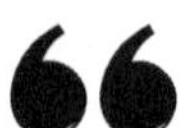

INSPIRING QUOTE

"Prayer is something exalted, supernatural, which dilates the soul and unites it to God." — Therese of Lisieux

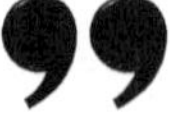

HEALING HINT

James Dillet Freeman's *Prayer for Protection* (1943 version) has been one of the most repeated and impactful lines of prayer verse in modern times:

The light of God surrounds me;
The love of God enfolds me;
The power of God protects me;
The presence of God watches over me.
Wherever I am, God is!

PRAYER

It's again important to emphasize that this section is referring to prayer — not religion and not related to attending religious services.

When we talk about prayer, it's much more in line with meditation or having a private conversation with a higher power. The praying we do in a church, synagogue, temple, mosque, or other places of worship is all good, but the one-on-one prayers have much more power in providing mental and physical health benefits.

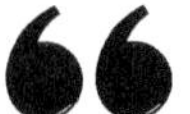

INSPIRING QUOTE

"In my deepest, darkest moments, what really got me through was a prayer. Sometimes my prayer was 'Help me.' Sometimes a prayer was 'Thank you.' What I've discovered is that intimate connection and communication with my creator will always get me through because I know my support, my help, is just a prayer away." — Iyanla Vanzant

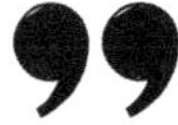

Several studies have shown a positive relationship between prayer and mental health. The results show that for many people, with prayer, they have:

- Fewer depressive symptoms
- Higher self-esteem
- Higher levels of life satisfaction
- Helped stay in recovery

AUTHOR INSIGHT

For me, one of the most powerful scripture verses deals with the beautiful outcome when we accept God (and the Holy Spirit) into our lives. In Galatians 5:22-23, the Apostle Paul discusses nine specific outcomes *("the fruit of the Spirit")* — love, joy, peace, forbearance, kindness, goodness, faithfulness, gentleness, and self-control — that result from the work of the Holy Spirit in a Christian's life.

These results make sense and are further validated by other research showing that prayer has a direct impact on the brain's production of serotonin (a chemical messenger — a neurotransmitter — that stabilizes mood, as well as feelings of happiness and well-being).

Furthermore, some suggest that prayer has a replenishing effect on serotonin and other neurotransmitters, creating an environment in which new brain cells are created, promoting brain health.

Finally, prayer is a vital tool many people use as a means to cope with everyday life and trauma history. It's an effective coping mechanism, with power for healing, but you might need to do more to heal than just pray. Prayer is not necessarily THE answer, but one of the tools.

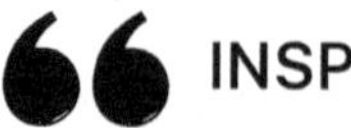

INSPIRING QUOTE

"Prayer is when you talk to God; meditation is when you listen to God." — Diana Robinson

A sample prayer for well-being/healing: Dear God. Thank you for this life and for supporting me even when I could not support myself. You give me so much love and hope to continue walking in faith for this life you have created for me. You are my Light. You are my Love. You light my darkness and warm me with love. I pray that you will continue to bless me and give me the mental fortitude to continue on my healing path. Amen.

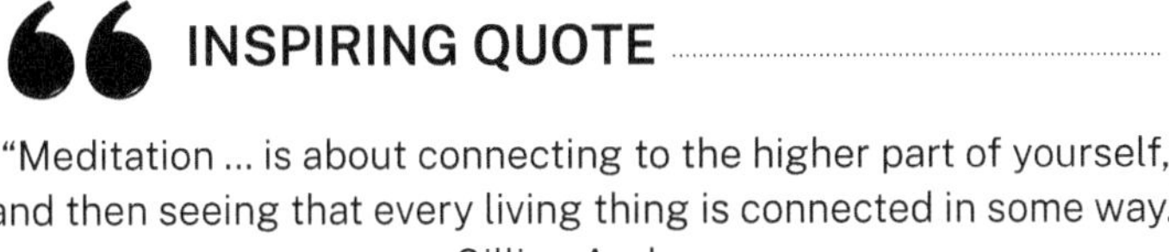

INSPIRING QUOTE

"Meditation ... is about connecting to the higher part of yourself, and then seeing that every living thing is connected in some way."
—Gillian Anderson

MEDITATION

Meditation is derived from the Latin *meditari*, which means "to think over, to consider, to ponder." More commonly, it refers to deep, often solitary reflection and thought.

Meditation is a great way to simply just **be**. To be fully in your body and mind, blocking out the many outside influences trying to reach your brain.

Benefits of meditation include gaining a new perspective, increasing self-awareness, reducing negative thoughts/feelings, increasing imagination and creativity, strengthening patience and tolerance, lowering blood pressure, and enhancing sleep quality.

More interestingly, though the research is not perfect, meditation also has other benefits in helping manage the symptoms of anxiety, depression, chronic pain, high blood pressure, irritable bowel syndrome, tension headaches.

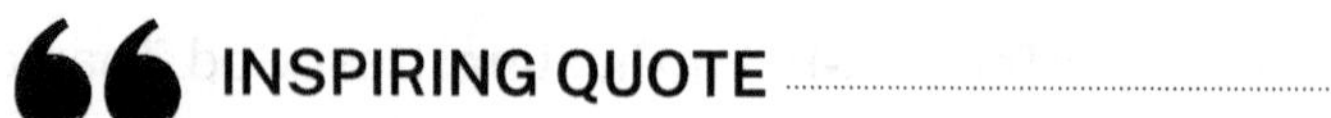

"Meditation is a vital way to purify and quiet the mind, thus rejuvenating the body." — Deepak Chopra

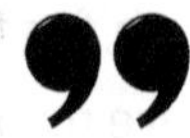

Emotional and Physical Benefits of Meditation

- Growing awareness of the connectedness of all things
- Improving brain plasticity
- Gaining new perspectives
- Building skills to manage your stress
- Increasing self-awareness
- Reducing negative emotions
- Increasing imagination and creativity
- Increasing patience and tolerance
- Enhancing sleep quality

Meditation can help manage symptoms of conditions such as:

- Anxiety
- Chronic pain
- Depression
- High blood pressure
- Irritable bowel syndrome
- Sleep problems

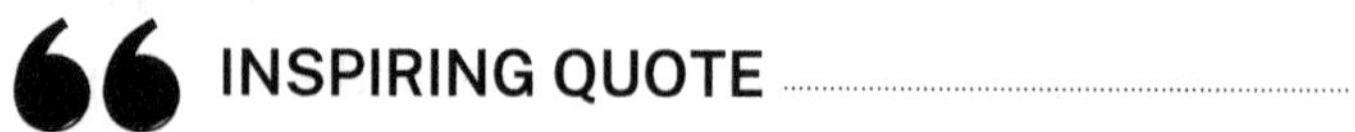

"Meditation is miraculous. Meditation should be a 'treatment of choice' for all of us — for healing trauma, building resilience, preventing illness, enhancing happiness, and prolonging life." — James S. Gordon, MD

Types of Meditations

1. Mindfulness Meditation — simply taking moments throughout the day to allow the world to stop spinning around us. Not necessarily a deep healing meditation, but one that helps us manage our days.
2. Spiritual Meditation — prayers of thanksgiving and gratitude for the blessing and grace received.
3. Mantra Meditation — using a word, phrase, or syllable that we repeat over and over again to block out distracting thoughts.
4. Guided Meditation — listening to the meditating instruction from a teacher who leads you through a session.
5. Gratitude/Love Meditation — a celebration of love and connectedness with each other and the Universe, with a focus on love, compassion.
6. Focused Meditation — about focusing thoughts on one of our senses, thus blocking out all other thoughts/feelings and concentrating on ONE thing.
7. Movement Meditation — combining the quieting of the mind with gentle movements of the body.
8. Transcendental Meditation — developed by Maharishi Mahesh Yogi, this style refers to a specific practice designed to quiet the mind and introduce a state of peace and calm.

Finally, remember the keys to meditation:

- Focused attention (to clear your mind of all the distractions)
- Relaxed breathing (to help calm your entire system)
- Quiet setting (to help stay focused and present)
- Comfortable position (to assist in staying in the meditation longer)
- Open attitude (to resist judgments, negative thoughts)

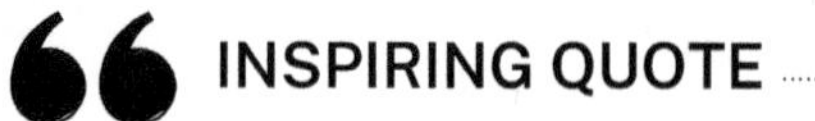

INSPIRING QUOTE

"Mindfulness is about being fully awake in our lives. It is about perceiving the exquisite vividness of each moment. We also gain immediate access to our own powerful inner resources for insight, transformation, and healing." — Jon Kabat-Zinn

MINDFULNESS

Mindfulness is about living in the moment, appreciating all the little moments in life that often get overlooked or ignored. It's about objectively observing our world — with grace, compassion, gratitude, acceptance.

Being "mindful" takes the work a bit deeper — to move toward a way of being (and we are Human Beings) in which our emotions, thoughts, and actions reflect a calmness and a focus on the present moment. The good news? Research suggests that obtaining a mindful brain can lead to a happier and more productive life.

While mindfulness is rooted in Buddhist and Hindu teachings, it does not have any religious aspects to it other than developing an appreciation for cherishing our time on this planet. Elements of mindfulness have been incorporated into several mental health practices, including Cognitive Therapy, Dialectical Behavior Therapy, and Acceptance and Commitment Therapy, among others.

The core elements of mindfulness are awareness and acceptance. Awareness of things happening in the present moment and acceptance of that awareness and any related thoughts. To be able to do these things, however, takes practice.

Key Elements of Mindfulness

What follows are some key aspects of mindfulness that should be explored and cultivated as you drop deeper into this practice.

1. **Being Fully Present.** We tend to live in a world in which we think we can multitask, but the reality is we can only do one thing at a time — it's called task-switching — and if we are going to practice mindfulness, the first thing we have to do is take ourselves off of autopilot and into the moment.
2. **Letting Go of Judgment.** Our goal, which we may not be able to accomplish initially, is simply to take on the role of an observer. It's learning we do not need to label everything we observe as good/bad, happy/sad, etc. We can simply observe and take note.
3. **Being Patient With the Process.** The key is trusting the process. You can certainly start mindfulness with an intention — such as being more aware of the moments in your day — but don't make that intention a goal you judge yourself against. It takes time to create new brain habits.
4. **Trusting Yourself.** Take note of your feelings, emotions, observations during your mindfulness, and trust your intuition about what you are observing. Trust in your abilities to make this practice something useful in your life.
5. **Acceptance.** As the observer, your goal is not to act or be a change-maker, it is simply to observe and accept what you see and feel.

Benefits of Practicing Mindfulness:

1. **Greater Gratitude.** We can often get caught up in the world around us, forgetting the gifts and beauty we possess; mindfulness brings us to the present, to a moment of reflection and gratitude.
2. **Stress Reduction.** We often live in an almost constantly "on" world, with deadlines, meetings, and more — all clamoring for attention; mindfulness slows the world down, brings calm and peace.
3. **Better Health.** We live in a world filled with chemicals, toxins, and other elements that can affect our health; mindfulness has been shown to help lower blood pressure, strengthen the immune system, improve digestion.
4. **Enhanced Creativity and Problem-Solving.** We often move from one project to another, non-stop; mindfulness forces us to stop, reflect, and perhaps find one or more new perspectives and solutions.
5. **Sharper Focus and Better Memory.** We can easily get caught up in the people and projects around us, losing focus on key issues; with mindfulness, we have the ability to focus and retain more.
6. **Enriched Sleep.** We are in a society in which sleep is sometimes elusive, as all the issues of the world seem to hit us as we lie on our pillows; mindfulness is the perfect tool for calming the mind and the body and preparing for a deep sleep.
7. **Improved Self-Esteem.** We are constantly being bombarded with messages about how we can be better, more successful, thinner; mindfulness has been shown to boost self-esteem, self-worth, and contentment with life.

8. **Happier Relationships.** We are social creatures, needing love and connections, and yet we often take so many of these relationships for granted; mindfulness helps us not only appreciate all the little things people do for us, it also helps us overlook/downgrade people's flaws and annoying habits.

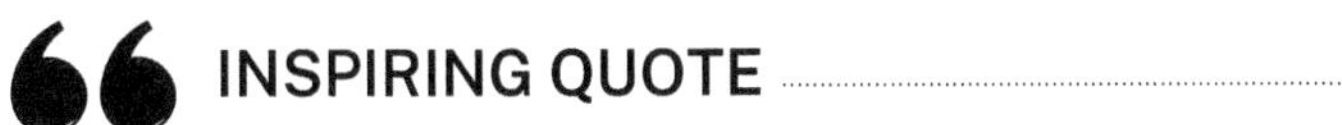

"Spiritual work and psychological work are both necessary to reclaim our true nature. Without psychological strength, spiritual practice can easily become another addictive distraction from reality. Conversely, shorn of a spiritual perspective we are prone to stay stuck in the limited realm of the grasping ego, even if it's a healthier and more balanced ego." —Gabor Maté, MD

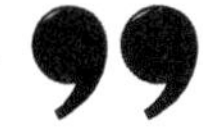

AFFIRMATIONS

Do you remember Stuart Smalley (played by comedian Al Franken), from the old *Saturday Night Live* skits? He was constantly looking in the mirror and repeating these words: "I'm good enough, I'm smart enough, and doggone it, people like me."

But he also said other things, such as "I deserve good things. I am entitled to my share of happiness. I refuse to beat myself up. I am an attractive person. I am fun to be with."

Humor aside, there's strong evidence of positive effects from using affirmations. The word affirmation comes from the Latin word *affirmare*, meaning to make firm, strengthen, or fortify. Self-affirmations are phrases that affirm our self-worth, often reflecting on our core values, which then allow us a broader view of the self—and our self-worth.

AUTHOR INSIGHT

For the past five years or so, my partner and I have used a set of affirmations — things we want to happen or accomplish — that we hang by our office workstations, making them easily accessible.

Some examples of strong affirmations:

- I am a good and amazing person. (self-confidence)
- I will find the perfect job for me. (self-confidence)
- I give permission to my brain to release what's not working for me. (healing)
- I am ready to release all ideas and feelings that no longer serve me. (healing)
- My body is healthy and strong. (health)
- I am worthy and deserve true love. (love/acceptance)
- I am talented and in demand. (self-esteem)
- I deserve to be happy. (happiness)
- I am doing the best I can. (acceptance)
- I am at peace. (acceptance/letting go)
- I am grateful for my life. (gratitude)
- I breathe in peace and harmony; I exhale stress and worries. (calm)
- Peace flows through my mind and body. (calm)
- Money flows freely to me. (wealth)

HEALING HINT

Words have power, and affirmations are a great tool to help avoid a lot of the negative self-talk that is often related to our traumas. We must avoid words like "can't," "never," "hate." Again, it's all about perspective and reframing the situation.

Interestingly, a recent study examined people who used affirmations with those who don't. The results demonstrated that people who practiced positive affirmations showed a higher level of activity in the regions of the brain that focus on self-worth. (Details here: https://www.ncbi.nlm.nih.gov/pmc/articles/PMC4814782/)

HEALING HINT

For people who are religious, affirmations can easily be part of daily prayers. You can also use an affirmation as your focus in meditation.

Finally, let's not forget about the ***Law of Attraction***, which states that whatever we can imagine in our mind's eye is achievable, but only if we act on a plan to get what we want. Furthermore, If we focus on negative thoughts and bad outcomes, we will attract them. If we focus on positive thoughts, have goals, and have a plan — then this is what will manifest into our lives.

Key Elements of the Law of Attraction:

- Positive Affirmations
- Gratitude Practice
- Visualization/Vision Boards
- Acting on Goals
- Surrendering and Accepting

HEALING HINT

If you are having trouble sticking to a schedule of spiritual healing/prayer/meditation, consider creating a sacred place in your home to serve as a makeshift "spiritual center." Make it so that it is only used for your healing purposes and you'll find it calming all the time.

HEAL ME WHOLE: UNDERSTANDING THE HEALING FROM SPIRITUALITY CHECKLIST

Here's a quick checklist for Chapter 4 to make sure you gleaned all the important points made about healing via spirituality in this chapter.

Remember to actually check off each of these to showcase your understanding!

- ☐ I realize that spirituality is bigger than any religion — and simply a belief that there is some higher power, something greater than us.
- ☐ I understand that spiritual healing can come from a number of different practices, including prayer, mindfulness, and meditation.
- ☐ I recognize the power of prayer, not only in connecting to my God, but also for the replenishing effect it has on serotonin and other neurotransmitters.
- ☐ I comprehend the many benefits of quiet meditation, including helping with anxiety, depression, chronic pain, high blood pressure.
- ☐ I get the function of mindfulness to put us into living in the moment, in the present, which often results in feelings of enhanced gratitude, joy, creativity, and memory.
- ☐ I know that while affirmations may seem a bit hokey, there is strong evidence for their use in promoting positive self-talk and helping eliminate negative self-talk.

CHAPTER 5:
Somatic Therapy & Body Healing

We are human *beings*, not human sloths. We are meant to be being!

This chapter is all about respecting your body, working your body, and releasing trauma from your body. We know trauma affects our entire body — and not just the mind.

You'll find a detailed discussion about somatics and exercise (yoga, dancing, walking, running, biking, etc.) in this chapter. Nutrition and nature also play a role in the body, but we'll add to this discussion in future chapters.

There are two key elements within this healing modality — specific body movements to help promote healing and the daily exercise that is important to maintaining good health and to stimulate healing.

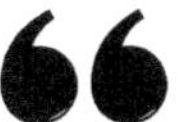

INSPIRING QUOTE

"Movement is a medicine for creating change in a person's physical, emotional, and mental states." — Carol Welch

PHYSICAL WAYS TO RELEASE TRAUMA:

- Laughing
- Tapping
- Dancing
- Shaking

- Bodywork/Massage therapy
- Walking
- Chakra balancing
- Sound therapy
- Yoga
- Somatics
- Exercise therapy
- Grounding
- Reiki

Many of these techniques are self-explanatory, but we'll take a closer look at several, including: bodywork, sound therapy, yoga, somatics, and exercising (for both health and healing).

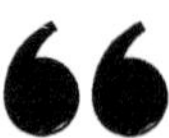

INSPIRING QUOTE

"Sound is vibration. It has power to affect us literally from the atoms up. Certain sounds, provided in the right context and combinations, can organize our neural activity, stimulate our bodies, retune our emotions." — Don Campbell

TAPPING

Tapping is a powerful tool based on the principles of ancient Chinese acupressure combined with modern psychology. It combines the cognitive reprocessing benefits of exposure and acceptance therapy with the energetic disturbance releases associated with acupuncture and other energy therapies.

Tapping is proven to reduce stress, lower cortisol, improve sleep, reduce anxiety, relieve pain, and increase productivity. More than 60 research articles report a staggering 98 percent efficacy rate with the use of this procedure from psychological distress

(PTSD, phobias, anxiety, depression) to physical conditions (asthma, fibromyalgia, pain, seizure disorders) to performance issues (athletic, academic).

Tapping helps regulate the nervous system and boost the immune system by putting the body back into the parasympathetic (relaxation) nervous system response. This allows the immune system, digestive system, reproductive system, and endocrine system to function as it should.

AUTHOR INSIGHT

One of the best pieces of advice I received from my psychedelic medicine coach was to use the tapping method during any challenging moments in my journey, tapping the Ren Meridian (also known as the Sea of Yin) near my heart at the sternum, and saying a mantra of "All is well; all is good." (Yin is the energy of relaxation and massaging this area helps release stress and find flow with the world.)

The key with tapping is releasing the bad stuff — the unprocessed trauma responses, the stresses, the pain — by saying or thinking about the issues you are trying to release. It's not a conversation, so just start and let the words come; they may not make any sense. If you're feeling nothing or numb, be sure to express that while tapping.

HEALING HINT

Think of tapping like someone hugging you during a scary moment; the physical sensation is sending a message to your body that it's all okay, eventually helping to reprogram your body into reacting differently to triggers.

There are two main tapping techniques — one using the meridian and one using chakras.

1. **Emotional Freedom Technique (EFT):** Uses the meridian system (like acupuncture), focusing on the meridian points — or energy flows and hot spots — to restore balance to your body's energy. Research shows that this method is good at rapidly reducing triggered emotional pain and distress. The key is balancing the energy flow in all areas of your body to maintain the best health; acupuncture uses needles to apply pressure to these energy points. EFT uses fingertip tapping to apply pressure. EFT is sometimes referred to as "emotional acupuncture" or "psychological acupressure."
2. **Chakra Tapping:** Use the chakra system (the seven major energy systems within the body; keep reading to learn more about chakras later in this chapter.) The problem is when chakras become unbalanced or closed, resulting in issues with corresponding nerve bundles and major organs. Thus, the goal with this tapping is clearing the stuck energy (stuck trauma responses). The process is the same as with EFT, but focused on 30 taps on each chakra, with or without statements of what you are hoping to clear.

HEALING HINT

Tapping has been shown to help combat veterans suffering from post-traumatic stress disorder (PTSD) — and should be great news for so many suffering with PTSD. The study found that after EFT treatments, the veterans had significantly reduced psychological distress and such a reduction in PTS that more than half no longer qualified as having PTSD.

Source: https://pubmed.ncbi.nlm.nih.gov/23364126/

BODYWORK/MASSAGE THERAPY

Think of bodywork therapy as massage therapy on steroids and with a specific focus. Massage therapists typically focus on soft tissue manipulation while bodywork goes much deeper.

Bodywork is a holistic approach to healing and treating pain — meaning that it is meant to treat all the parts of the body, mind, and spirit.

Bodywork involves manipulation techniques for eliminating muscle tension, increasing range of motion, and realigning the entire body so that it can move without pain. It involves some massage elements, but also often includes breathwork, visualization, and emotional release techniques.

Bodywork therapists can often incorporate other healing methods, such as Reiki, acupressure, and reflexology.

Some common types of bodywork:

- Rolfing. Fixing posture by aligning the connective tissue in the body.
- Craniosacral: Relieves symptoms from different physical and mental health conditions, such as migraines, depression, and more.
- Feldenkrais Method: Movement-based therapy to help build and increase body awareness.
- Alexander Technique: Helps with improving posture and movement by aligning head, neck, and body.
- Hellerwork: Combines body movement education with manual therapy to realign the body, helping eliminate stress.

- Neuromuscular: Involves soft tissue manipulation to improve the function of the nervous system and the alignment of the skeletal system.
- Tension & Trauma Releasing Exercises (or TRE®): a simple yet innovative series of exercises that assist the body in releasing deep muscular patterns of stress, tension and trauma. Created by Dr. David Berceli, Ph.D.

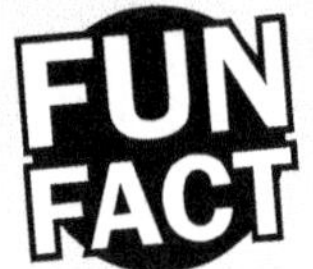

While most people focus on the 7 major chakras in the body — crown, third eye, throat, heart, solar plexus, sacral, and root — others believe we may have 114 different chakras in the body!

CHAKRA BALANCING

There's a unique system of energy flow and spiritual power in our bodies sometimes referred to as "spiritual energy," and it flows into the cells, tissues, and organs of our bodies. This is not some supernatural concept, but a way for us to examine the different aspects of wellness in our emotional and physical bodies.

HEALING HINT

The flow of energy through our chakras is strongly affected by our personalities and our emotions, as well as our state of spiritual development. The more trauma we hold, the more blockage exists in our energy flow through the chakras.

We have seven major energy systems in our bodies known as chakras, which comes from the ancient Sanskrit word for "wheel," and some healers claim they look like spinning wheels of color and light. Each chakra has a different function and color, with each one being associated with a specific element and physical organ in the body. The chakras run along the length of our spines — and end at the top of our heads.

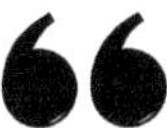

INSPIRING QUOTE

"Each of the seven chakras are governed by spiritual laws, principles of consciousness that we can use to cultivate greater harmony, happiness, and well-being in our lives and in the world." — Deepak Chopra

These chakras are affected by our personalities, our traumas, and our state of spiritual development — and it is extremely important that these energy centers are balanced. The goal is to have a balanced energy system, otherwise it can lead to illness, stress, anxiety, depression.

Chakra balancing does not require being an expert or belief in the supernatural. At a basic level, the chakras can be seen as metaphors for different aspects of our wellness in our emotional and physical body.

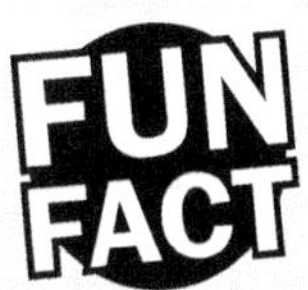

When you have cleared all your chakras, it allows Kundalini energy to flow. Kundalini is considered to be a life-force energy. We all have it, but not all of us have experienced it as a spiritual "awakening." When the Kundalini energy is flowing, old problems and even past trauma do not have the same effect on you anymore. You remember them, but they no longer bother you.

The Primary Chakras:

1. Root: Base of spine; color is red. Associated with the will to live, life-force, survival, fear-safety issues, fertility, stability
2. Sacral: Just above pubic bone; color is orange. Associated with sexuality, vitality, enjoyment of life, creativity, self-esteem, ethics

3. Solar Plexus: Upper abdomen; color is yellow. Associated with self-image, power, self-esteem, willpower, strength, fear
4. Heart: Just above the heart; color is green. Associated with emotions, unconditional love, loneliness, peace, sympathy, forgiveness, trust, compassion, spiritual development
5. Throat: The throat; color is blue. Associated with self-expression, communication, creativity, self-discipline
6. Third Eye: Between the two eyes on forehead; color is indigo. Associated with intuition, inner vision, inspiration, spiritual awakening, telepathy
7. Crown: Very top of the head; color is violet or white. Associated with spiritual awareness, consciousness, grace, wisdom, connection to *Higher Self*

When energy becomes blocked in a chakra, it triggers physical, mental, or emotional imbalances that manifest in symptoms such as anxiety, lethargy, or poor digestion.

Balancing chakras is the process of tending to these areas of your body and thoughts so that you may feel more aligned, authentic, and healthy. It's something that can be done on your own, but it's also something that can be accomplished through sound therapy, meditation, yoga, reiki... even a walk in nature.

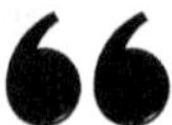

INSPIRING QUOTE

"Much of the healing you experience in a sound bath is of your own making. You are the catalyst for your own change, and it's you who creates the magic of the experience." — Sara Auster

SOUND THERAPY

Sound is everywhere and it's part of our waking lives — and sometimes even when we're sleeping.

If you've ever been to a concert or listened to music on a powerful speaker, you know the power of music to affect our bodies, our minds, our moods — and that's the rough theory behind sound therapy. Sounds affect the mind, body, and soul.

But it also interesting to note that we spend a large portion of our lives unaware of the sounds that surround us.

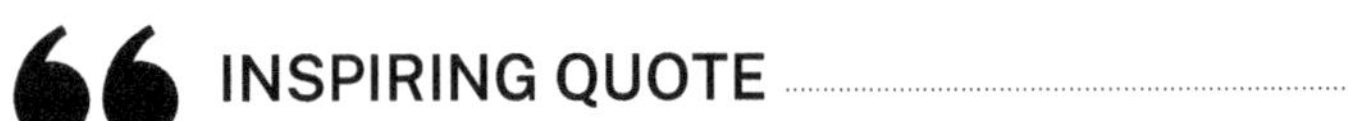

INSPIRING QUOTE

"Since the human body is over seventy percent water and since sound travels five times more efficiently through water than through air, sound frequency stimulation directly into the body is a highly efficient means for total body stimulation, especially at the cellular level." — Jeffrey Thompson.

As holistic healing has spread, sound therapy has gained traction — and some are stating that this therapy can help with improved focus, decreased physical pain, and enhanced mood. Sound therapy has the ability to ease, energize, and empower us!

There's limited, but growing research on this therapy. One study from the University of California found that meditation aided by Tibetan bowls noticeably decreased stress and anger — especially among people who were new to this kind of practice.

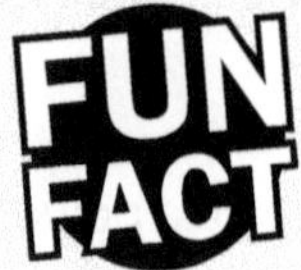

Sound therapy is just one form of "vibrational" healing. Another is light therapy. All forms of vibrational healing deal with rates of frequency and vibration. Your body's chakra energy centers are also associated with a specific color — and colored lights, stones, or cloth are often used to balance these centers. (Red, blue, and full spectrum light are the most commonly used colors for healing with light.)

Furthermore, University of Bonn researchers found evidence among 30 separate studies that support the use of binaural beats as a way to reduce anxiety. Finally, scientists from McGill University examined 400 studies and found that playing and listening to music improved overall mental and physical health.

Finally, we also know that playing upbeat music typically causes the blood vessels to expand, improves breathing patterns, and stimulates increased production of endorphins — while decreasing stress and increasing a sense of well-being.

Sound therapy uses a variety of sounds and music and covers a range of treatments, from music therapy to sound baths. It has been used for thousands of years to realign the body's vibration and improve mental health issues and emotional well-being.

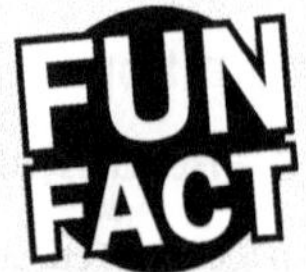

Like so many other therapies, the key to healing is the intention. Setting an intention to heal is so vital to moving forward with your healing.

Types of Sound Therapy:

- Sound baths (uses instruments like crystal bowls, gongs, tuning forks, and chimes to initiate a full-body listening experience)
- Music therapy (uses therapist-guided vocal sounds and chants to enhance memory and alleviate stress)
- Binaural beats (involves playing two separate tones in each ear, which are perceived as a single, almost euphoric tone by the brain. (Other forms of sound therapy work much in the same way.)

One thought is that the vibrations from the sounds or music have a massaging effect that permeates our entire body. As with so many other healing modalities, you get from this therapy what you desire; YOU are the catalyst for healing.

Reported Benefits From Sound Therapy:

- Enhanced mental health/outlook
- Better sleep and relaxation
- Decreased pain and inflammation
- Reduction in headaches
- Better joint movement
- Disappearance of kidney stones

YOGA

Yoga is a fantastic form of mental and physical exercise that has been used for centuries. The overall philosophy of yoga is about connecting the mind, body, and spirit... an integration of all layers of life, including environmental, physical, emotional, psychological, and spiritual.

It is an ancient spiritual practice that originated in India, but yoga has become quite Westernized and modified. The key to yoga is the work of pairing breath and movement together. It is an expansive collection of different spiritual techniques and practices aimed at integrating mind, body, and spirit to achieve a state of enlightenment or oneness with the universe.

And guess what? Unlike many other types of exercise, almost anyone can start practicing yoga. For those with some physical issues, such as being overweight or recovering from an injury, it's best to start with a gentle practice; after you've built up the strength and flexibility for more challenging sequences, you can simply enhance/elevate your yoga practice.

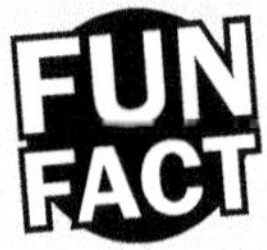

According to the book, The Seven Spiritual Laws of Yoga, "your body is a field of molecules; your mind is a field of thoughts. Underlying and giving rise to your body and your mind is a field of consciousness — the domain of the spirit."

Scientific studies show that the regular practice of yoga and its postures may help to stimulate the body's endocrine glands and metabolism. Furthermore, the more yoga you do, the better your physical endurance and the more you strengthen your resistance to illnesses.

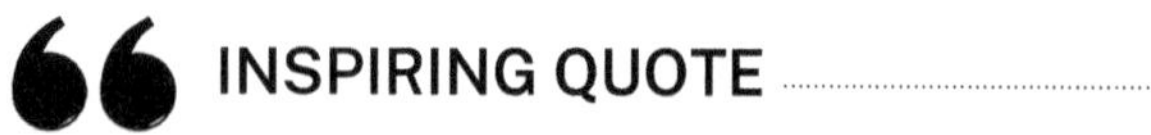

INSPIRING QUOTE

"Yoga is the journey of the self, through the self, to the self." — The Bhagavad Gita

There are yoga studios everywhere, including online, and you need very little equipment to get started with yoga: a yoga mat so

that you're comfortable with the movements and some clothing that can stretch and move freely with your body.

Key Benefits of Yoga:

- Improve flexibility, stamina, mobility, posture, and balance;
- Increase muscle tone and strength;
- Improve/maintain well-being, reduce depression;
- Strengthen mind-body connection;
- Reduce stress/promote relaxation;
- Boost the immune system;
- Maintain/lose weight;
- Helps improve sleep;
- Prevent medical/health conditions.

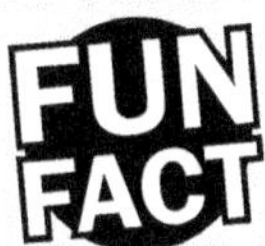

Yoga can be traced back to northern India more than 5,000 years ago.

Branches of Yoga:

- Yama: Deals with rules of social behavior, the core of yoga: practicing nonviolence, speaking truthfully, exercising sexual control, being honest, and being generous.
- Niyama: Deals with rules of personal behavior (how you live/act when no one is watching), and includes: purity, contentment, discipline, spiritual exploration, and surrendering to the Divine.
- Hatha: What most Westerners practice, which combines the practice of asanas (yoga postures) and pranayama (breathing exercises), with a goal of supporting an inward, introspective awareness — bring peace to the mind and body.
- Raja: A stricter form, which focuses on mind and body control.

Raja means royal, and this practice is for attaining enlightenment through meditation and energetics.
- Karma: Is about attempting to reach a point of selfless service through unselfish, kind, and generous actions; goal is to attain enlightenment.
- Bhakti: Has a focus on cultivating acceptance and tolerance; the goal is to reach the state of rasa (essence), a feeling of pure bliss achieved in the devotional surrender to the Divine.
- Jnana: Focuses on wisdom, the path of the scholar, and developing the intellect through study; to become liberated from the illusionary world of maya (self-limiting thoughts and perceptions).
- Tantra: About transforming one's physical, mental, emotional, and spiritual body into one unified whole; the pathway of ritual, ceremony, or consummation of a relationship.
- Bikram: Consists of the same, copyrighted twenty-six postures and two breathing techniques, in the same order for ninety minutes, in a room heated to 105°F (40.6°C), with a humidity of 40%. Sometimes referred to as "hot yoga."
- Kundalini: Incorporates repeated movements or exercises, dynamic breathing techniques, chanting, meditation, and mantras. It is designed to awaken the energy at the base of the spine in order to draw it upward through each of the seven chakras.
- Integrative Yoga Therapy (IYT): Brings together multiple yoga techniques (asanas, pranayama, mudra) along with mantras and meditations for therapy, as a healing art.

Yoga maintains that chakras are center points of energy, thoughts, feelings, and the physical body.

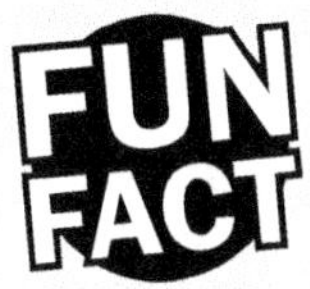

Traditional talk therapy focuses on cognitive or thinking skills, known as the top-down method. Somatic therapies focus first on the body, known as a bottom-up approach.

SOMATIC THERAPY

Somatic therapy is any holistic psychotherapeutic process that incorporates mind-body exercises and other physical techniques (such as dance, massage, grounding, breathwork, meditation) related to the mind-body connection; it can also include talk-therapy as part of the healing.

It's designed to help you understand yourself and your body — and the signals your body transmits about areas of pain, discomfort, or imbalance... trauma. It can help heal from past traumas and help prepare for managing future stress.

As you might have guessed already, somatic simply means "relating to the body." Somatic therapy is all about helping the release of pent-up trauma that has become "trapped" in the body.

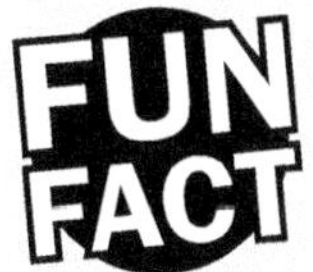

Humans possess a somatic nervous system, which allows us to move and control muscles throughout our body. It also feeds information from four of our senses — smell, sound, taste, and touch — into our brain.

Amazingly, studies have shown that somatic therapy can effectively treat post-traumatic stress, with one study showing that 44 percent of participants lost the diagnosis of PTSD following treatment.

HEALING HINT

Grounding (sometimes referred to as earthing) is a therapeutic technique that involves doing activities that "ground" or electrically reconnect us to the Earth, allowing electrical charges from the Earth to have positive effects on our body. Find more information about grounding for health here: https://www.healthline.com/health/grounding-techniques

Dr. Thomas Hanna, an educator in the field, coined the term *somatic* in 1970 to describe several techniques that share one important similarity: They help people increase bodily awareness through a combination of movement and relaxation. That same decade, Dr. Ron Kurtz developed the Hakomi Method, which combines somatic awareness with experiential techniques to promote psychological growth and transformation.

While somatic practices have become increasingly popular in the Western world over the last 50 years, many of them draw from ancient Eastern philosophy and healing practices, including tai chi and qi gong.

Somatic therapy techniques include:

- Body awareness
- Grounding
- Movement
- Self-regulation
- Acting out physical feelings
- Stillness/calmness
- Emotional releasing through sequencing
- Developing new physical tools

Somatic therapy is especially good in helping with:

- Grief
- Anger
- Anxiety
- Depression
- Chronic pain
- Stress
- Trust
- Intimacy
- Insecurity
- ADHD

HEALING HINT

Somatic therapy helps bring awareness to where trauma is stored in the body, thus giving people the tools to release the trauma, whether through mindfulness or mindful exercises such as yoga or tai chi.

Types of Somatic Therapy:

- Hakomi Method
- Massage/Bodywork therapy
- Acupuncture
- Chiropractic work
- EMDR
- Neurosomatic therapy
- Myofascial release
- Craniosacral therapy
- Polarity therapy
- Somatic experiencing
- Sensorimotor psychotherapy
- Yoga

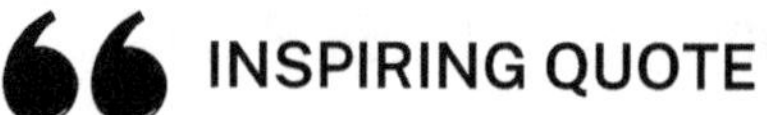

INSPIRING QUOTE

"Exercise is king. Nutrition is queen. Put them together and you've got a kingdom." — Jack LaLanne

EXERCISE THERAPY

Somehow, we have even managed to get exercise wrong!

Every January, we witness a huge jump in gym memberships, only to see them go down again in the ensuing months.

Exercise should not be an ideal or something we strive for. Instead, we should think of exercise as fun, and good for our overall health — mental, physical, emotional, spiritual.

We know regular exercise helps boost your brain functioning, elevate your mood, increase feelings of positivity, and help deal with depression, anxiety, and stress. And because the body and soul are connected, taking care of your body helps boost spirituality as well.

HEALING HINT

Research studies show that exercise can treat mild to moderate depression as effectively as antidepressant medication and counseling — without ANY of the side effects. Read more here: https://neurosciencenews.com/exercise-depression-medicine-22762/

Exercise on physical health: Regular exercise improves cardiovascular health, reduces body fat and blood pressure, lowers tension and stress, and increases energy levels, while also improving fitness, balance, sleep, and heart health in the long run.

And if you can combine some of that exercising with time in nature? Double win. In fact, studies show outdoor activities like hiking, sailing, mountain biking, rock climbing, whitewater rafting, and skiing have also been shown to reduce the symptoms of depression and PTSD.

Why do so many of us seem to dread exercise? Again, I think it's because we simply have the wrong concept of it. It's not like we have to devote hours of our days to exercising. Research studies indicate that ***modest*** amounts of regular exercise can make a big difference in our overall health — regardless of age, fitness level, experience.

A recent British study found that if everyone simply completed 11 minutes of daily exercise — such as ***vigorously*** walking, hiking, biking, swimming, stair-climbing, dancing, yoga, playing tennis, etc. — one in 10 premature deaths could be prevented.

"You should feel yourself moving, your heart will beat faster but you won't necessarily feel out of breath," says Dr. Soren Brage, who led the research. The findings show that this amount of exercise is enough to reduce the risk of developing heart disease and stroke by 17 percent and cancer by 7 percent.

Sadly, even at just 11 minutes a day — equating to only a little more than 1 hour (75 minutes) weekly — the researchers concluded that few people accomplish that minimum of exercise.

AUTHOR INSIGHT

You have to find the exercise (the physical activity) you enjoy most — and do it at a time that fits you. Years ago, I decided roller-blading in the early mornings was going to be my thing, but I started in the fall, and it became impossible to get up early enough to do it. I switched to biking, including biking to work most days, and found everything worked for me. Find your favorite way to exercise.

Furthermore, in a review of all the literature, results show that simply doubling that time commitment to just 150 minutes each week (about 20 minutes a day) of various types of vigorous physical activity (such as brisk walking, lifting weights, biking, and yoga) ***significantly*** reduces depression, anxiety, and psychological distress, compared to traditional treatments, such as antidepressants and benzodiazepines and anxiolytic medications.

Benefits of Exercise:

- Boosts mental health
- Increases physical health
- Improves energy levels
- Promotes better sleep
- Weight management
- Strengthens sexual arousal
- Can enhance social interactions

As a side note, if you are not able to complete vigorous exercise, you can get similar health benefits by simply doing a weekly routine that includes roughly 150-300 minutes of physical activity that raises the heart rate... thus, a 30-minute daily walk would accomplish this target. (Household cleaning and yardwork also count.)

Strength training too. It's recommended that adults also do activities that strengthen muscles twice a week. Yoga, Pilates, lifting weights, heavy gardening, and carrying heavy shopping bags all count.

Why does exercise seem to be so effective at helping maintain good health? When we exercise, all kinds of changes in the brain start happening, including neural growth, reduced inflammation, and new activity patterns that promote feelings of calm and well-being.

Exercise also releases endorphins, powerful chemicals that energize your spirits and make you feel good. Finally, exercise can also serve as a quiet and peaceful distraction, helping break any cycles of negative thoughts that feed depression.

Finally, while I feel most people can fit some sort of exercise into their daily lives, another UK study found that people who can only exercise on the weekends had almost the same health benefits as those who exercise daily — so go be your full-on weekend exercise warrior. Do NOT make up excuses not to exercise — it is so beneficial to healing... and health.

For the physically disabled, exercise is often more challenging, but not impossible — and the health benefits are worth the extra effort. Remember that the key is movement and resistance, and whether your disability is temporary or permanent, there are trainers and other resources that can guide you. One place to start is with this article, Top 10 Exercises for Disabled People (https://disabilityhorizons.com/2016/10/top-10-exercises-disabled-people/)

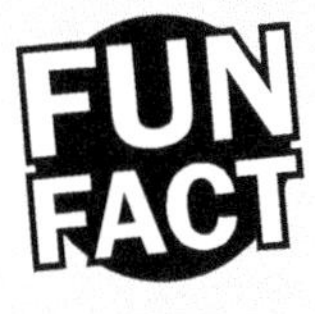

Several recent studies have found that people who have walked outside report a higher level of vitality, enthusiasm, pleasure and self-esteem, and a lower level of tension, depression, and fatigue. Furthermore, people who exercise outside also say they are more likely to exercise again than those who stay indoors.

REIKI

Reiki is energy work that utilizes the chakra system as a guide for healing and centering of the entire self: mind, body, and spirit. It is thought that energy can stagnate in the body where there has been physical injury or emotional pain; if not treated, these energy blocks can cause illness.

Reiki is a Japanese term meaning "energetic spirit." *Rei* is a general term for universal spirit, while Ki is about energy, vitality, life force. (People have actually been practicing forms of Reiki for more than 2,500 years.)

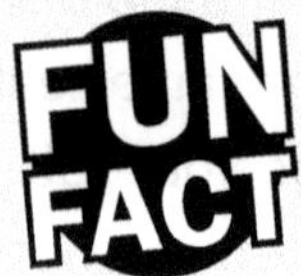

The concept of energy as spiritual life force can be seen by different names in many cultures: Prana (India), Chi (China), Mana (Polynesia), Nyama (West Africa), Orenda (Iroquois), Waken (Lakota), Ruach (Hebrew), and Barraka (Islam), Aura (Russia), Chu'lel (Mayan).

Healing is all about balancing the energy flow in your body, bringing harmony to your chi, or life force energy. It promotes relaxation and reduces stress and anxiety through gentle touch. Reiki practitioners use their hands (sometimes without even touch) to deliver energy to your body, improving the flow and balance of your energy to support healing, and unlocking your chakras.

The current form of Reiki is a fairly new practice, developed in the early 1900s.

Reiki is known to foster feelings of:

- Wellness
- Peace
- Relaxation
- Security

INSPIRING QUOTE

"The Reiki method is not only for curing illness. Its true purpose is to correct the heart-mind, keep the body fit, and lead a happy life using the spiritual capabilities human beings were endowed with since birth." —Mikao Usui

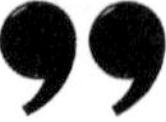

Reiki is a great tool for relaxation, stress reduction, and symptom relief. It can:

- Encourage physical, emotional, mental, and spiritual healing
- Foster healing after injury/surgery
- Stimulate the immune system
- Promote natural self-healing
- Relieve pain and tension
- Bring on a meditative state

Reiki differs from other touch therapies, such as massage, in that there is no pressure, massage, or manipulation involved. You may experience a feeling of energy moving through you, with sensations like heat, tingling, or pulsing.

Very little scientific research has been conducted on Reiki, but anecdotal evidence suggests that it may induce deep relaxation, help people cope with difficulties, relieve emotional stress, and improve overall well-being.

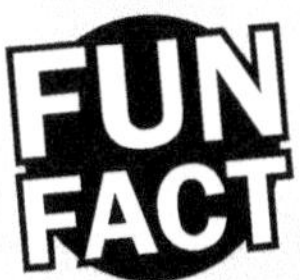

Reiki is a practice that anyone can learn, and it can be used on oneself as well as others. Once you have learned the basic techniques, you can begin practicing Reiki on yourself. It is important to find a quiet, comfortable place to do Reiki, as this will help you to relax and focus your energy.

While Reiki is about healing the whole body, people have used this healing method for several ailments, including:

- Back pain
- Heart disease
- Chronic pain
- Depression
- Anxiety

- Cancer
- Autism
- Fatigue
- Neurodegenerative disorders

Reiki Principles:

- Just for today, I will give thanks for my many blessings.
- Just for today, I will live consciously in the moment.
- Just for today, I will not worry.
- Just for today, I will not be angry.
- Just for today, I will do my work honestly.
- Just for today, I will be kind to my neighbor and every living thing.

Finally, it should be noted that it usually takes several weeks to adjust to a Reiki attunement. During that time, you may have intense dreams and experience detoxification symptoms (such as runny nose, diarrhea, increased urination). It's simply a process of energy adjustments; you will still feel well.

HEALING HINT

Acupuncture, the ancient Chinese art of needling the body to produce healing, is another potential tool in your body-healing toolbox.

HEAL ME WHOLE: UNDERSTANDING THE HEALING FROM SOMATICS CHECKLIST

Here's a quick checklist for Chapter 5 to make sure you gleaned all the important points made about healing via somatics and exercise in this chapter.

Remember to actually check off each of these to showcase your understanding!

- ☐ I realize that there are multiple physical ways to release trauma, including laughter, yoga, tapping, dancing, grounding, and more.
- ☐ I understand that physical healing methods are important for assisting in my healing journey, as well as in maintaining my healing.
- ☐ I recognize the power of bodywork — of physical manipulation of my body and the energy fields within my body — in healing.
- ☐ I comprehend the power of sound to impact mood, but when combined with intention and other healing techniques (such as meditation or prayer), it can be a powerful tool for healing.
- ☐ I value the many healing benefits of yoga — for both physical strength and healing, as well as for the spiritual and mental components.
- ☐ I know that somatic therapy (including Hakomi, grounding, movement, self-regulation, acupuncture, EMDR, and more) can help with all sorts of healing, including bringing awareness to where trauma is stored in the body.
- ☐ I recognize the value of exercise — for physical health, better brain functioning, and increased feelings of positivity... as well as for helping deal with depression, anxiety, and stress.

CHAPTER 6:
Nature Healing

Our Indigenous ancestors knew the importance of nature; they lived, gathered, and hunted in nature. Furthermore, for thousands of years, humans turned to nature to help heal their ailments—using flowers, stems, bark, and roots to heal mental, physical, and spiritual ailments.

We are not meant to spend our entire lives cooped up in homes and offices; we are meant to be outside, enjoying the many benefits, from breathing fresh air, to the beautiful scents, to the gentle sounds, to the powerful life-enhancing chemicals plants release, to the Vitamin D we absorb, to the health benefits and reduced stress.

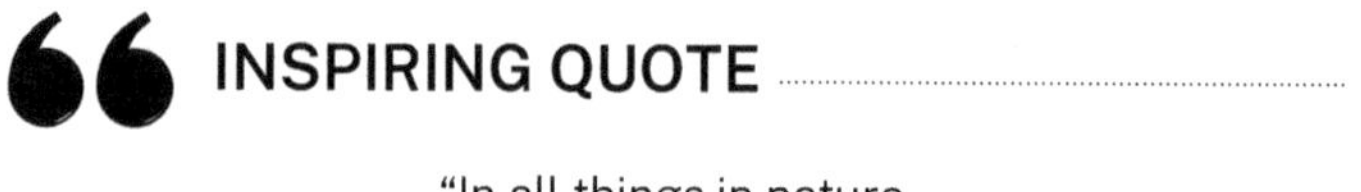

"In all things in nature,
there is something of the marvelous." —Aristotle

The Japanese have a practice of walking through forests as a way of reducing stress. Called *shinrin-yoku*, which roughly translates to "forest bathing," it involves opening the senses to the woody aroma of the trees and other plants, the green scenery, and the soothing sounds of streams and waterfalls... because they know all of these elements play a part in promoting better health and well-being.

I have known for years of the power of nature to heal. Just getting outside to the sights and scents of nature is enough to lift my spirits and brighten my day. It is one thing to feel the healing powers and another to read the scientific research that builds a very strong case for the life-saving, life-enhancing, nature of nature.

HEALING HINT

Research is abundantly clear: nature is not only nice to have, but it's a must-have for physical health and cognitive function. Nature is essential to our health.

And you don't have to travel miles to your local national forest or wilderness; the research shows it works just as well as when you sit on a bench in your neighborhood park — or even just your backyard. Spending any time outdoors can help positively impact our health (physical, mental, spiritual), but especially during stressful times — and even simply when taking a break from electronic screens.

AUTHOR INSIGHT

Besides working in our forested property most of the year and gardening in the summer months, my partner and I also spend as much time as possible on our deck in the warmer months... out in nature, focused on mindfulness and gratitude, soaking up Vitamin D from the sun, listening to birdsongs (and an occasional healing podcast, lol).

FIVE WAY NATURE HELPS HEAL US

1. Nature Helps Fight Depression, Relieve Anxiety. Nature is awe-inspiring for many people, but not surprisingly, research has found that being out in nature has even more profound effects. A study published in the *Proceedings of the National Academy of Sciences* reported that subjects who walked for 90 minutes in a natural area, such as a forest or nature park, had lower activity in an area of the brain associated with depression than people who walked in urban areas.

Nature, at a minimum, seems to lift people's spirits, say the authors of the study, but negative ions — oxygen atoms with an extra electron — found in forests may also contribute to reducing depression symptoms. For example, in a typical building, there are less than 100 negative ions per cubic centimeter, but near a waterfall such as Yosemite Falls, negative ions can easily exceed 100,000 per cubic centimeter.

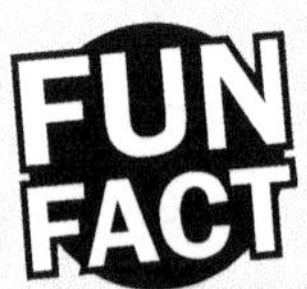

The Japanese have a beautiful word: *komorebi*; it literally means "sunlight leaking through trees," or, "dance between shadow and light," which is perfect for describing the beauty when rays of light dapple through overhead leaves and shine through to the ground. It's also interesting in relation to wellness, as we go through periods of struggle (darkness) and wellness (light).

2. Nature Reduces Premature Mortality. One study found that exposure to parks, forests, and other green spaces was associated with reduced mortality from stroke, cardiovascular disease, and diabetes among older adults.

Furthermore, other studies clearly show that nature helps reduce stress hormones, including adrenaline and cortisol. Nature helps calm the fight-or-flight mechanism. This research is especially important for people suffering with post-traumatic stress. We know that living with long-term stress is a killer, leading to a long list of complications.

HEALING HINT

Here's why time in nature rocks! Western medicine tries to imitate what is already in nature through synthetic drugs that can be patented, and they always come up short. That's why pharmaceutical drugs come with a laundry list of side effects (including death!) — and nature and natural remedies have few.

3. Nature Helps Lower Blood Pressure. If you are one of the 1 in 3 Americans affected by high blood pressure, taking time to venture out into nature has been shown to be good for your heart. A large-scale study at the University of Queensland, Australia, found that about 10 percent of people with high blood pressure could get it completely under control without medications if they simply spent 30 minutes or more in a park at least once a week.

Besides the tranquility and improved air quality of natural spaces, some scientists also believe that the phytoncides trees release lowers blood pressure by repressing the body's flight or fight response, which stresses the body... as well as reducing the stress-related hormones cortisol and adrenaline.

4. Nature Promotes Cancer-Fighting Cells. Having lost both parents to cancer, and knowing how many people die annually from cancer, I need to believe in the power of nature to help ward off cancer. Happily, studies are supporting this theory.

A study at Nippon Medical School found that when people walk through a forest, they inhale those phytoncides from the trees — which then increase the number of natural killer (NK) cells; these NK cells are a type of white blood cell that supports the immune system, which are associated with a lower risk of cancer. NK cells are also known for fighting inflammation, which has a role in many major health issues.

Monthly forest walks could be an important lifestyle factor in the prevention of cancer as well as helpful therapy for people diagnosed with cancer.

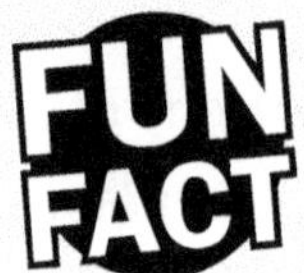

Ecotherapy is an approach based on the idea that people have a deep connection to their environment and to the Earth itself. In this same line of thinking, failing to nurture this connection can take a toll on your well-being, particularly your mental health.

5. Nature Helps With Attention-Deficit Disorders. Short trips into nature can help improve concentration and attention. A study at the University of Michigan found that people improved their short-term memory by 20 percent after a nature walk... and another study at the University of Illinois at Urbana-Champaign discovered that children with ADHD who took a 20-minute walk in a park (without their medications), were able to concentrate much better after the nature walk.

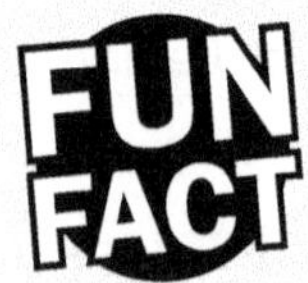

Are you a nemophilist? It's someone with a love or fondness for forests, woods, or woodland scenery, or someone who often visits them — a 'haunter' of woods. The word derives from the Greek *nemos*, meaning grove, and *philos*, meaning affection. One who is fond of the forest.

6. Nature Promotes Cognitive Functioning. Studies show time spent in nature helps restore human psychology, promoting recovery from mental fatigue and improving cognitive functioning — through a process called "Attention Restoration

Therapy," coined by Rachel and Stephen Kaplan in their book, *The Experience of Nature.*

Combine walking and nature, and the results are even more interesting. In a University of Michigan study, researchers found that participants who walked in nature for 50 minutes performed significantly better in cognitive functioning than those who walked the same amount of time in an urban setting.

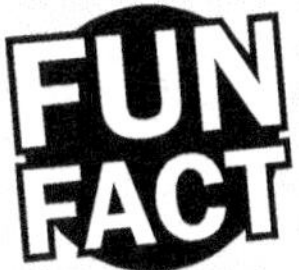

Research shows that even if the elements of nature are artificial, the images, sounds and smells of nature can have positive health effects. For example, people listening to nature sounds through headphones felt a sense of calm.

7. Nature Promotes Spiritual Connection. Evidence shows that people get a greater sense of the vastness of nature and the universe when spending time outdoors, which often leads to feelings of gratitude to a "higher power" for creating the planet.

Many people combine time spent in nature with prayer or meditation, further deepening that spiritual connection to the *anima mundi*—the soul of the world, the living spirit of creation. Some believe that unless we make a relationship to the soul of creation, we are just scratching the surface of life.

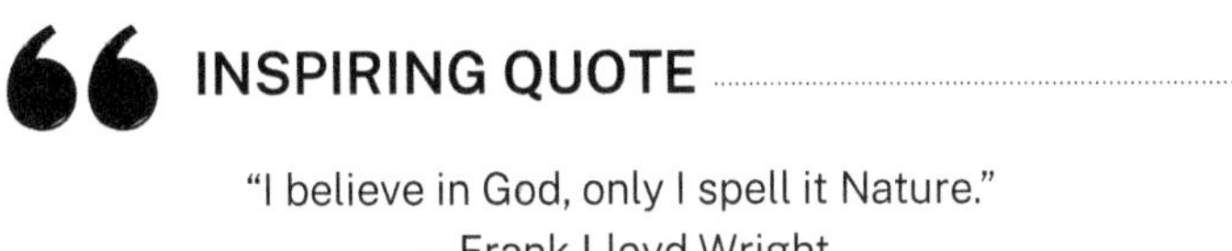

"I believe in God, only I spell it Nature."
—Frank Lloyd Wright

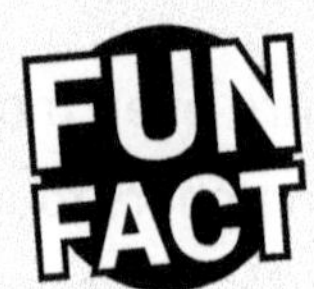

While you're out in nature, don't be afraid to get your hands or feet dirty! Studies show that a non-pathogenic organism — *mycobacterium vaccae* — lives in soil and is a "friendly bacteria" and supportive of our health. In fact, some researchers theorize one reason for the rise in allergies and autoimmune diseases in industrialized countries is because most of us no longer farm — no longer spend time working in the dirt.

WHAT ARE PHYTONCIDES?

Phytoncide is a substance released by trees (and other plants) and generally means the aroma of the forest. *Phyton* means "plant" in Latin, and *cide* means "to exterminate."

Phytoncides play an important role in tree/plant immunity, and are produced to help trees protect themselves from harmful insects and germs.

What are you waiting for? Get out in nature today! Make it a habit to spend 30 minutes daily basking in the glory and healing powers of nature... naturally.

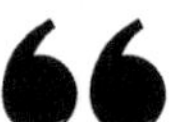

INSPIRING QUOTE

"I go into nature to be soothed and healed and have my senses put in order." — John Burroughs

PREPARING FOR TIME IN NATURE

You're not going to get all the benefits of time in nature unless you follow a few simple guidelines.

1. **Release Any Expectations/Rules.** You are out to engage with nature, but other than that goal, don't have any other expectations... and definitely do not put a timer on your healing.

2. **Strive For Two Hours Per Week.** A recent study of 20,000 people found that two hours a week spent in a natural setting — either in one sitting or with the time spread across the week — resulted in participants good health and psychological well-being.
3. **Keep Your Screen Away.** The whole point of being in nature is to get away from technology, distractions, social media, etc.
4. **Engage All Your Senses.** The best part of time in nature is how everything seems better, brighter. The colors are brighter, the sounds fascinating, the scents powerful.
5. **Find a Place to Sit — and BE.** Many people walk or hike in nature, and that's fine, but make sure you take time to just sit IN nature and absorb it all.
6. **Consider Small Supplies.** If you plan to spend a fair amount of time in nature, you might want to bring layers of clothing, as well as water and a healthy snack.
7. **Keep Practicing.** For very active people, it might be hard to just be still in nature, but that's exactly what forest bathing is all about. So, keep practicing until you find peace.
8. **Find a Guide.** If you feel like you need a little guidance on this whole forest-bathing thing, consider hiring a professional guide. One such organization that offers guides is the Association of Nature and Forest Guides and Programs (https://www.natureandforesttherapy.earth/)

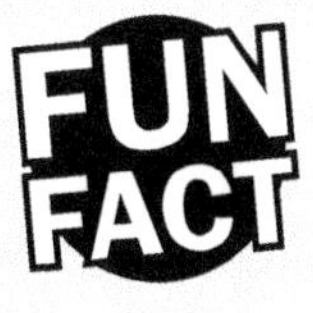

An increasing number of organizations are also embracing the back-to-nature paradigm. One organization, Park Rx America, has as its mission "to decrease the burden of chronic disease, increase health and happiness, and foster environmental stewardship, by virtue of prescribing nature during the routine delivery of healthcare by a diverse group of health care professionals."

HEAL ME WHOLE: UNDERSTANDING THE HEALING FROM NATURE CHECKLIST

Here's a quick checklist for Chapter 6 to make sure you gleaned all the important points made about healing via nature in this chapter.

Remember to actually check off each of these to showcase your understanding!

- ☐ I realize spending time in nature offers many benefits, including Vitamin D from the sun, phytoncides from the trees, and a reduction in stress levels.
- ☐ I understand that people have been using nature for healing for centuries, including the Indigenous and the Japanese, with their practice of "forest bathing."
- ☐ I recognize any amount of nature helps; I do not need to travel miles to a national park or forest. Spending time in my backyard or city park also provides the same benefits.
- ☐ I comprehend nature promotes calmness of mind while also helping with improved cognitive functioning.
- ☐ I get that nature helps strengthen a spiritual connection — and that many people pray or meditate in nature, offering gratitude for this amazing planet.

CHAPTER 7:
Breathwork

Most of our breathing is done at the subconscious level; it's one of the body's automatic systems. We never have to think about our breathing and we probably never really even notice it except for times when we are out of breath.

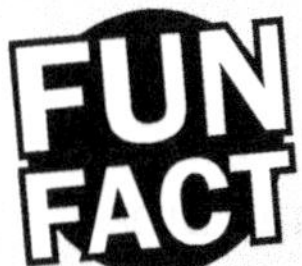

In the yoga tradition, the breath is said to carry a person's life force. The breath is considered a conduit of life. It is the physical manifestation of your chi — or lifeforce energy — and you do it 23,000 times a day.

Breathwork is about bringing our breathing to the forefront. It's about actively engaging our breathing, and it is probably the most undervalued and underutilized tool for dealing with trauma. More and more people are using this technique for improving physical, mental, emotional, and spiritual health.

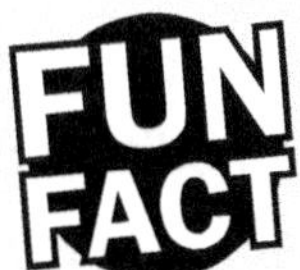

There are many types of breathwork techniques; some from ancient practices, such as Pranayama, and others, modern techniques developed by doctors and other practitioners.

Breathwork is used in meditation and yoga, but it is also a category all unto itself. It's about bringing us right into the present moment, to be actively engaged with ourselves. It's a tool to help regain focus and put healing in the forefront.

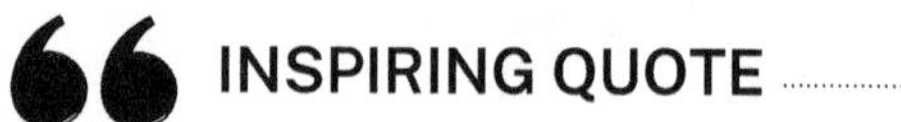

"If I had to limit my advice on healthier living to just one tip, it would be to simply learn how to breathe correctly." — Dr. Andrew Weil

By incorporating breathing exercises into your daily routine, you may be able to get rid of several pills and supplements you're currently taking, including antidepressants, anti-anxiety pills, painkillers, statins, antiacids, sleeping pills, and many more.

SCIENTIFIC BENEFITS OF BREATHWORK:

1. **Improves Mood and Self-Esteem... and Healing.** Breathwork helps us improve our moods, build our self-confidence, enhance our self-image, and foster greater self-love... and push away negative thoughts and feelings.
2. **Allows Us to Focus on Our Trauma.** When we use breathwork with intention to get into a relaxed state of being, it allows us to examine our trauma from a safe place. Furthermore, people can hire a breathwork coach to help with advanced methods for healing.
3. **Helps Manage Depression.** When breathwork is combined with other healing methods, such as yoga or meditation, it can help alter your mood (to one of calmness), ground you, and assist in your gratitude practice.
4. **Reduces Stress and Anxiety.** These structured breaths can help you take back control of your fight-or-flight response following stressful situations, bringing peace and calm.
5. **Helps Manage Pain.** Breathwork can help manage pain, especially chronic pain (which may or may not be caused by trauma); researchers have found that these breathing

techniques help enhance feelings of relaxation, taking the focus away from the pain.

6. **Boosts Health and Immunity.** Because you bring in more oxygen when doing breathwork exercises, you are actually contributing greatly to your overall health. Breathwork alkalizes our blood and calms our sympathetic nervous system, which can help lower our systematic inflammation.
7. **Lowers Blood Pressure.** Using slow and deep breathing exercises helps activate your parasympathetic nervous system, which will help decrease your heart rate and dilate your blood vessels, which then helps reduce your blood pressure.
8. **Improves Sleep.** One of the most direct benefits of breathwork is help with sleep. Studies show that breathwork is perhaps the best natural sleep aid, helping lower energy levels and reducing all the chatter in your brain.
9. **Helps With Digestion.** If you struggle with digestive issues (including constipation, diarrhea, or IBS), breathwork may help improve your digestion by getting more blood circulating (which actually helps improve ALL of your body's systems).
10. **Improves Focus and Creativity.** Instead of popping a pill for focus, try breathwork. Research shows that breathwork helps people with poor focus. Furthermore, because breathwork helps you clear your mind and relax, it allows your brain to make new connections, increasing creativity.
11. **Enhances Spirituality.** Using some of these breathing techniques can result in a mystical experiences and deep spiritual insights. The word "spirit" is derived from the Latin word *spiritus* which literally translates to "breathing; breath; breath of a god."

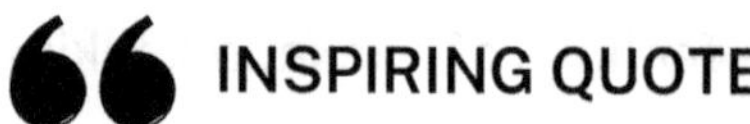

INSPIRING QUOTE

"Breathing affects your respiratory, cardiovascular, neurological, gastrointestinal, muscular, and psychic systems, and also has a general effect on your sleep, memory, ability to concentrate, and your energy levels." — Donna Farhi

The good news is that you don't need any equipment or special props or tools to start a breathwork practice. And, at least in the beginning (and depending on your goals), doing breathwork may only take 5 minutes out of your day. As you go deeper, your time spent with breathwork will likely increase.

Types of Breathwork Techniques:

- **Deep Breathing.** The simplest breathwork technique involves inhaling through your nose for a count of four, holding it in for a moment, and then exhaling slowly out through your mouth until you've emptied all the air from your lungs.
- **Box (Square) Breathing.** Popularized by Navy Seals and the military, it involves 4 x 4 counts (like the perimeter of a box); inhaling through the nose for a count of four, holding it in your lungs for a count of four, exhaling through the nose for a count of four and then holding again for a count of four.
- **Holotropic Breathwork.** Uses breathing patterns that take you to an altered state of consciousness, where you can address your physical, emotional, and spiritual pain. The goal here is to breathe rapidly to induce an altered state, with *holotropic* meaning "moving toward wholeness in oneself." (Created by transpersonal Czech psychiatrists Stan and Christina Grof.)

- **Conscious Energy Breathing.** This practice is about breathing in energy, as well as air. It involves using "circular breathing," quick, shallow breaths without any breaks between an inhale and an exhale. Also referred to as Rebirthing Breathwork, and developed by Leonard Orr in the 1970s.
- **Pranayama Breathwork.** Consists of structured breaths, and positively affects the autonomic nervous system, which controls essential functions of the body like the heart rate, respiration, and blood pressure. The name comes from *prana*, meaning "the universal life force," and *ayama*, which means "to regulate or lengthen."
- **Shamanic Breathwork.** Focuses on the use of breathing techniques to release the inner healer within you. It begins by establishing a safe and sacred space through various rituals and ceremonies such as smudging with sage. You then lie down and focus on surrendering to your inner shaman. (Developed primarily by Linda Star Wolf in the 1990s.)
- **Transformational Breathwork.** The goal here is to find your inner-healing center, and involves taking deep in-breaths and then letting the air out — without controlling the out-breath. The work is often done with a facilitator who can help locate tension spots.
- **Wim Hof Breathwork.** Based on the ancient pranayama method, his method involves using breathwork: taking thirty power breaths, followed by taking a deep inhale and retaining your breath as long as comfortable, then exhaling. Afterward, one must inhale deeply for another 10-15 seconds, retain, and then exhale.
- **Circular Breathing.** This breathwork can release old emotions, cleanse the energetic and emotional body, and even

open up the mind to deep spiritual insights. It involves taking a gentle breath in and out without pausing.

- **Visualization Breathing.** The key aspect of this breathing technique is combining it with a visualization of affirmation. Some ideas:
  - Visualizing pain, depression leaving your body with every deep exhale;
  - Visualize breathing in light, breathing out darkness;
  - Visualize light washing your body of darkness as you inhale and exhale;
  - Visualizing each of your seven chakras healing as you breathe into them;

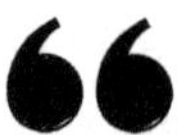

INSPIRING QUOTE

"Deep breathing is the tool of the masters for letting go of old attachments and old emotions and for extracting the wisdom hidden within the experiences of life." — Ron Teeguarden

HEAL ME WHOLE: UNDERSTANDING THE HEALING FROM BREATHWORK CHECKLIST

Here's a quick checklist for Chapter 7 to make sure you gleaned all the important points made about healing via breathwork in this chapter.

Remember to actually check off each of these to showcase your understanding!

- ☐ I understand that breathwork is about bringing us to the present and being actively engaged with ourselves.
- ☐ I realize that breathwork techniques offer opportunities or healing and the reduction of medications and painkillers.
- ☐ I recognize that I can start breathwork without any special tools or training — and the benefits can be realized with just 5 minutes per day.
- ☐ I get that multiple breathwork techniques exist, from things like deep breathing to shamanic breathwork to the Wim Hof Method... and I need to find the ones that work best for me.
- ☐ I comprehend that breathwork can be combined with several other holistic methods, such as yoga and meditation.

CHAPTER 8:
Nutrition

If you're like many in the Western world, what you're eating is most likely contributing to your poor health — physically and mentally. To combat the overwhelming misinformation being fed to us (pun intended), we have to take matters into our own hands, which means committing more time and energy into what you buy and eat.

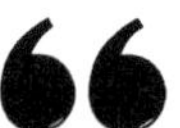

INSPIRING QUOTE

"What science is revealing is that people who adhere to a protocol that's rich in healthy, anti-inflammatory fats and proteins enjoy significantly lower rates of depression. Conversely, a diet high in carbs and sugar is fanning the flames of inflammation." — Kelly Brogan, MD

For our overall health and well-being, we **need** quality foods and safe liquids. Our nutritional plan must include high-quality, nutrient-dense ingredients that will be a key source of metabolic fuel to power our cells, organs, and nervous system.

The sad state of farming in the U.S. — and in many parts of the world — is that the vast majority of farming is now conducted by large agribusinesses, not farmers; these businesses destroy the soils of nutrients and routinely spray toxic chemicals (fertilizers, insecticides) on the crops. Many also use GMO seeds.

Furthermore, many of the foods we buy are prepacked and processed/refined, with many of the nutrients naturally found in the raw ingredients removed by all the processing techniques. Not convinced? Search "hyperpalatable foods" and you'll be shocked at food producers are doing to our food.

AUTHOR INSIGHT

I won't admit to how many times I trauma-ate ice cream or cake or chips... all my bad comfort foods. And guess what? Those crappy foods may have given me temporary happiness in those moments, but they wreaked havoc on my health and impeded my healing. What we eat *REALLY* matters.

Because of the poor soil quality and the overuse of the same crops (monoculture), the food we eat today — even the good, organic stuff — is simply not as nutrient-dense as even a generation ago. Thus, most of us need to supplement our diets with vitamins and minerals.

Whenever possible, try to also source your primary foods locally. Doing so supports your neighbors who are farmers and ranchers, your food will be at its peak freshness, and you can talk directly with the farmers about how they produce their fruits, veggies, and meats. If you can't source locally, then please buy organic — mainly for the reduction of the amount of pesticides in your body.

Finally, just a mention about water. It's critical to health, but the water you're drinking might not be helping as much as you would like. Even municipal water systems can have contaminants, parasites, and chemicals in them. My suggestion is to obtain a quality water filter system; we use a Berkey and love it.

HEALING HINT

One of the key vitamins we are deficient in is Vitamin D, which is known to support both immune health and emotional health. This little vitamin may be a key piece in reducing depressive episodes, including in children. (Learn more here: https://pubmed.ncbi.nlm.nih.gov/28914205/)

DR. RANDALL'S 10 NUTRITION TIPS FOR HEALTHY LIVING & HEALING

Are you ready to live your best life? Are you ready to ditch the fad diets? Are you ready to make a lifestyle change?

I ask because many Americans have a pretty bad diet — and this is regardless of whether you are Keto, Paleo, Carnivore, Vegetarian, Vegan, or following some other fad diet. We even have a name for it: The Standard American Diet, or SAD.

What is the SAD? It consists of eating calorie-dense and nutrient-poor foods and beverages from factory farming and ranching that have been overly processed, contain added sugar and salt, produced with toxic fats and oils... and which sadly includes many of the brands you can find in the grocery store as well as in most fast foods.

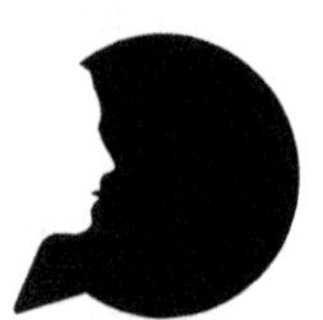

AUTHOR INSIGHT

I have been on a wellness journey for more than 20 years and rarely get sick; I took an extended trip this year in which I had to eat the SAD at restaurants and lodges for three weeks; I rarely had fresh fruits or vegetables and none of the food was organic — or local. The end result? Not only did I get sick, but amazingly, caught Covid for the FIRST time. Food can INDEED be medicine. Food/nutrition matters.

People on the SAD also eat minimal amounts of fresh fruits and vegetables, as well as few whole grains and legumes.

The unfortunate outcome of the SAD is that more and more Americans are overweight to the point of obesity — some studies say about 60 percent are obese — which in turn leads to other health issues, including:

- Inflammation
- Autoimmune disorders

- Cardiovascular (heart) disease
- Stroke
- Cancer
- Kidney and gallbladder issues
- Hypertension (high blood pressure)
- Diabetes
- Sleep apnea
- Depression
- Infertility

Stop eating yourself to death and make a few simple changes to your cooking/eating lifestyle. Here's the trauma-freeing, healing-first formula for eating.

HEALING HINT

Dr. Kelly Brogan discusses in her book, *A Mind of Your Own*, that many studies of the "Western" diet "demonstrate that a diet marked by processed vegetable fats, sugar, preservatives, and a battery of other chemicals may be setting us up for the development of chronic inflammation."

1. Quit the Diets; Focus on Lifestyle

Diets don't work — and just about everyone on Earth could probably tell you that. I mean, some will help you lose weight initially (and perhaps with questionable safety), BUT they never work long-term because of feelings of deprivation and social isolation they can cause.

Are you one of the many Americans who are on a specific diet? Sadly, you are going to be disappointed, because even when diets are initially successful, lost weight is frequently regained within a few months.

Focus on a balanced lifestyle, eating from the rainbow of real foods, using the information and resources from the next 9 tips.

2. Stop Eating Processed Food

Processed foods are any food that has been altered from its natural state — by the manufacturer adding preservatives, flavorings, sweeteners, salt, fats/oils, and/or stripping away all the nutrients of the original ingredients. A good rule of thumb: If you can't pronounce an ingredient, you have no reason buying the product. Another rule? Don't purchase any premade item that has more than five ingredients listed on the label.

Examples of highly processed foods include pasta sauces, salad dressings, cake mixes, crackers, chips, deli meats, and all frozen and premade meals (such a pizzas and microwavable meals). Almost all fast foods are overly-processed to make them extra desirable to consumers.

Whenever possible, cook/bake from unprocessed, natural ingredients.

HEALING HINT

We have known the many dangers of processed (industrial, granulated) sugar for more than five decades; the way we consume it, it is hazardous — a "poison" — for our general health (obesity, diabetes, inflammation) and a cancer risk. (Read more here: https://www.theguardian.com/society/2016/apr/07/the-sugar-conspiracy-robert-lustig-john-yudkin)

3. Eliminate Processed Sugar and Simple Carbohydrates

The U.S. has the HIGHEST consumption of sugar in the world... on average, every (unaware) American consumes about 126 grams of sugar daily, which equates to about 100 pounds of added sugar per year. Scientific studies show the connection to addiction, obesity, heart disease, diabetes, cancer from sugar usage.

Where does all this sugar come from? From just about every item in the grocery store — and the sad part is that none of these items needs the added sugar. Thus, this change might be the hardest to accomplish because refined sugar (and its many other names) is in almost all processed foods you find in the grocery store — and not just the obvious sweet/dessert items like cookies and cakes and sodas and juices — including catsup, tomato sauce, salad dressing, bread, cereal, protein bars, yogurt, granola, soup, vegan milks and creamers, crackers, peanut butter, canned fruits, barbecue sauce, and mayonnaise.

HEALING HINT

Because of the poor quality of our soils and our foods, most people really should supplement with a high-quality multiple vitamin and a few others, including Fish Oil/Omega-3, Vitamin A, Vitamin C, Vitamin D3/K2, Vitamin E, Iron, Zinc, Magnesium, Turmeric/Curcumin. If you're not eating yogurt or other similar foods, you should also consider a quality probiotic for gut health. Consult with your doctor; or better, with a holistic nutritionist — because many supplements are also made of "filler" ingredients and/or poorly sourced (many from China) ingredients.

4. Consume Quality (Organic) Food

Many people have misconceptions about the organic label — other than the universal agreement that organic often costs a bit more than non-organic.

Products that are certified organic are made with foods that are (generally) grown/raised free of toxic pesticides and herbicides (such as Roundup), growth hormones, sewage sludge, and irradiation. No genetically modified organisms (GMOs) can be used.

Just eliminating the pesticides, herbicides, and antibiotics should be enough to have you buying organic — even if it means cutting back on other purchases... organics are an investment in your health and the health of your family. These toxic elements found in conventional foods are linked to increased levels of cancers, tumors, brain damage, and other health issues.

AUTHOR INSIGHT

One of the systemic problems we face in trying to improve the nutrition and diet of ALL people is the issue of food deserts: areas that have limited access to affordable and nutritious food — typically concentrated in low-income and historically marginalized areas (including inner cities and Native American reservations). Learn more here: https://foodrevolution.org/blog/food-deserts-food-oasis-healthy-food-access/

5. Eliminate All Bad Seed Oils

Did you know that most of the cooking oils used by Americans are actually ***bad*** for you? These industrial vegetable "seed oils" can cause a variety of conditions, including inflammation, heart disease, autoimmune issues, exhaustion, mental fog, weight gain, anxiety, mood problems, migraines, and headaches — according to Dr. Catherine Shanahan (aka Dr. Cate). She states: "Cutting out vegetable oils is the most powerful dietary change you can make."

These toxic seed oils are used in just about all fast food and other restaurant offerings, packaged foods, and home cooking and baking. More infuriating, several of these oils have been touted as "heart-healthy" when in fact, they are the opposite — full of chemicals/solvents from processing, as well as trans-fats and Omega-6 fatty acids.

Here's the list of **seed oils to avoid**: vegetable, canola, corn, cottonseed, sunflower, grapeseed, soybean, and rice bran.

Use these **good oils** instead: avocado, coconut, olive, and ghee (from grass-fed cows).

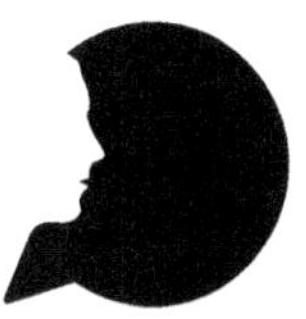

AUTHOR INSIGHT

Many experts believe coconut oil is a superfood — and it can certainly be used in many forms and in many ways. We have used coconut oil in cooking and baking, but mostly we take a daily capsule to make certain we are getting the benefits. Read more about the reasons you should be doing the same: https://draxe.com/nutrition/coconut-oil-benefits/

6. Buy From Local Ranchers and Farmers

Buying local is a win-win-win... a win for you because it will be the freshest food you eat (besides stuff you grow in your own garden); a win for your neighboring farmer or rancher; and a win for the environment, as many products are transported for thousands of miles to reach your local store.

Buying local can also be a fun and educational experience — getting to know your farming and ranching neighbors and learning more about how the food you are buying is raised and harvested. Many consumers have become disconnected from where their food comes from and how it is produced, but buying locally changes that — and hopefully influences people to start paying more attention to the foods they eat.

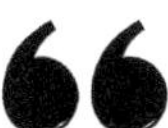

INSPIRING QUOTE

"Eat the rainbow! Include a variety of foods and flavors in your diet to improve satiety and boost your nutrition."
— Eliza Savage, MS, RD

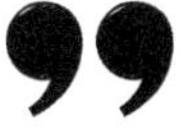

7. Drink Lots... of Water

Did you know that we often snack on food when we're actually thirsty but don't realize it? Water is your body's principal chemical component — and makes up more than half of your body weight. Your body depends on water to survive.

AUTHOR INSIGHT

I found that especially in the summer months, I need to consume electrolytes in about half of all the water I consume because I am susceptible to muscle cramps. There are several high-quality brands that do not use sugars to sweeten, including Ultima and LMNT.

Water is essential to good health. Lack of water can lead to dehydration, and even mild dehydration can drain your energy and make you tired.

According to the U.S. National Academies of Sciences, Engineering, and Medicine, men should drink about 15.5 cups of fluids daily while women should consume about 11.5 cups daily. These recommendations cover fluids from water, other beverages, and food — but excluding alcohol.

HEALING HINT

Chronic inflammation is a killer; it is when your body overreacts to a problem — and instead of moving in, healing the problem, and then returning to normal, the inflammation persists over time. A chronic state of inflammation can lead to numerous health problems, including heart disease, stroke, arthritis and joint disease, autoimmune disorders, depression, dementia and Alzheimer's disease, osteoporosis, and even cancer. More and more, we are discovering that systemic chronic inflammation is the common bond linking most chronic conditions.

8. Consider One Big Meal: Linner

Americans typically eat way more food daily than needed to function, survive. Most folks typically eat three big meals, plus unhealthy snacks, with sugary sodas, and wonder why they are gaining weight.

Here's what we do in my household: Coffee and a light snack in the morning; our main (healthy) meal in the early afternoon, which we call linner; and a light (and healthy) snack in the early evening.

Sometimes referred to as One Meal a Day (OMAD), this strategy is not so much a diet but rather a particular version of intermittent fasting — and simply avoiding overeating.

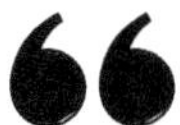

INSPIRING QUOTE

"Make healthy eating an easy choice by meal prepping when you have extra time. This can help make meal times or snacks quick, easy, and nutritious when you are short on time throughout the week." — Holly Klamer, MS, RDN

9. Meal Prep: Plan for Leftovers

One of the biggest hurdles people face with healthier eating and cooking from scratch is meal-planning, especially for busy families, but please remember you do not need to create extravagant meals like the people on so many cooking shows.

I simply don't understand the issue when people say they do not have the time to cook, as most of my meals take no more than 30 minutes to prepare and cook; bigger meals take longer, but I can also use a crockpot and other devices. Plus, while the initial big meal may take longer to prep, you should be able to get at least one other meal from it; sometimes, with a roast, I get three or four meals from one prep.

With just a small amount of planning, you can easily cook from scratch (or reheat those meals) 7 days a week.

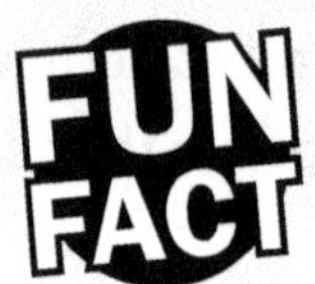

Why not include more eggs in your meal planning? Eggs are truly a superfood (especially when you can obtain them from a neighbor or local farm). We often have eggs as our main meal, sometimes as breakfast revisited and sometimes in the form of omelets and quiches. Learn more about the superpower of eggs: https://www.healthline.com/nutrition/why-are-eggs-good-for-you

10. Don't Forget the Fruits, Veggies, and Nuts

Most of us do a really poor job with eating enough fruits, veggies, and nuts.

In the summers, I grow and buy a lot of fresh fruits and veggies. I eat a lot, but also freeze portions to last until the next growing season. I freeze, but there are other options, such as canning. You can also buy (organic) frozen fruits and veggies. In the summers, we mostly drink our fruits and veggies in smoothies.

We also always have nuts on hand... for baking and for snacking. We add nuts in most of our baked goods and enjoy pistachios and macadamia nuts to snack on.

HEALING HINT

Many of us deal with trauma through stress eating, so the first step is recognizing your food cravings may be a result of being triggered—where you seek comfort through food (so-called comfort foods). Once you clear your trauma, food should simply become food again.

 INSPIRING QUOTE

"Eating clean, whole foods changed *everything* for me and my family; we feel great every day. The energy and mental clarity have been remarkable. I have eliminated many nagging symptoms I was dealing with, and dropped weight and inches. *I think I forgot what it felt like to feel good,* I was used to walking around bloated and inflamed." — Gerry Daniel

HEAL ME WHOLE: UNDERSTANDING THE HEALING FROM NUTRITION CHECKLIST

Here's a quick checklist for Chapter 8 to make sure you gleaned all the important points made about healing via nutrition in this chapter.

Remember to actually check off each of these to showcase your understanding!

- ☐ I recognize that in order to eat well, I need to spend much more time analyzing labels, changing my food shopping habits.
- ☐ I understand that the Standard American Diet (SAD) should be avoided, as should mass-produced meats and vegetables — which are grown/raised in bad conditions and often treated with chemicals, antibiotics, and hormones.
- ☐ I know I need to get my mind off the concept of diets and dieting and onto the idea of a healthy lifestyle, eating nutrient-dense real foods.
- ☐ I get that most fast foods and processed foods contain ingredients that are bad for me. Further, I realize that I should not be buying foods that contain ingredients I can't pronounce.

- ☐ I comprehend that I need to clean up my pantry by removing or greatly reducing my use of bad oils, sugars, and basic/simple carbohydrates.
- ☐ I grasp the importance of water and hydration and plan to drink more throughout the day.
- ☐ I acknowledge that organic and high-quality, locally-raised foods are probably my best choices for eating "clean" and healthy meals.

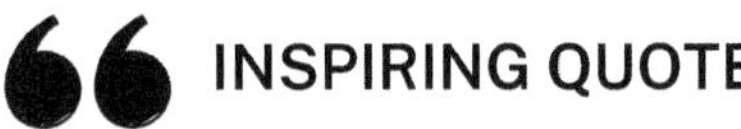

"A healer's power stems not from any special ability, but from maintaining the courage and awareness to embody and express the universal healing power that every human being naturally possesses." —Eric Michael Leventhal

PART TWO:

HOW TO FIND TRUE COACHES/HEALERS

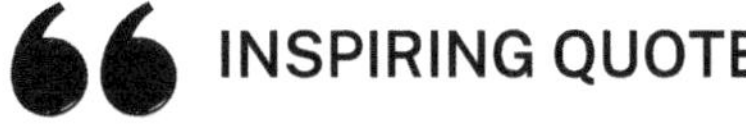

"I realized a while back that I have an innate ability to be compassionate, and I saw that the strength of compassion is something that healers have and healers use." —Ricky Williams

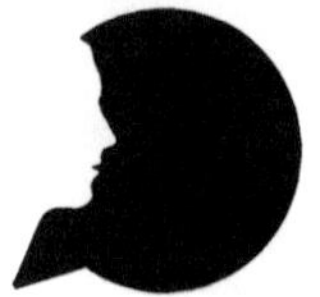

AUTHOR INSIGHT

The following pages contain advice and tips for finding holistic healers and coaches, written by experts in the fields. All good advice, all of which should be read. That said, it's also been my experience that once you find one good holistic doctor/coach/healer, they can refer you to others that they respect and trust — making it easier to find the additional healing modalities you seek.

CHAPTER 9:

How to Find a Holistic Nutrition Coach, from Randall Hansen, Ph.D.

Are you on a path to healing? Are you seeking an experienced expert to help you understand food and nutrition better?

Nutrition is not taught in schools much and even medical schools don't teach it; add all the confusing claims of the many diets and food-based fights (plants vs. meats) AND the misleading information on the foods we buy because of weak labeling laws — and it's no wonder many of us struggle with this key component of our health and healing.

A holistic nutrition coach can help you in multiple ways — helping to improve your understanding of the different types of foods and their impact on your health, focusing on any medical concerns/issues you may have, and providing you with a mature relationship with food and eating. Beyond food, these coaches may also assist you with tips for exercise, sleep patterns, stress reactions, and more.

It doesn't matter where you are on your healing journey, but if you have never thought about nutrition — or have been too focused on diets — then a nutrition coach might be the perfect choice for you.

To me, the key is finding a truly holistic nutrition coach; a coach who focuses first on you, second on your entire self (not just what you eat), and third on natural methods of healing.

When you conduct a search, the best keywords would be holistic nutritionist or holistic nutrition coach. You could also try holistic dietician, holistic health coach, holistic integrative coach. If you don't keep the holistic as part of your search, you will run into too many dogmatic coaches focused more on their own programs than on one designed specifically for YOU.

What To Look For in a Holistic Nutrition Coach:

- **Credentials and Training.** There are quite a few organizations that offer education and training in nutrition, but it's important that your coach has some formal training in nutrition, health. Note that the term nutritionist is not regulated, which means it's your responsibility to review credentials.
- **Philosophy.** While most true holistic coaches should be focusing on each client's needs, some coaches are more dogmatic than others — focused on a specific diet or specific foods — and you'll want to make sure your coach's approach matches your goals/lifestyle.
- **Testimonials from Past Clients.** The greatest insights about a coach can come from previous client testimonials, so request them if they are not readily available on the coach's website. Look for insights about the coaching style, approach, and success.
- **Program/Coaching Costs.** While health and healing should be our utmost priority, costs will always play a role in our decision-making. See what makes sense to you. If you are in deep need of understanding nutrition, then make the investment in a coach. If you're lucky, your health insurance may cover some of the costs.

- **Level of Support.** You'll find coaches that only do individual coaching and others that do group sessions. Some will only do in-person coaching while others are open to distance/telehealth coaching. The key is finding a coach with the level of support you need, want, desire.
- **Fit.** If you're like me, I only work with people who get me — and who are a good fit for my quirky personality. Thus, make sure you speak with each coach you are considering so that you can get a good feel for their personality. Why hire someone you don't like — or who doesn't get you?
- **Red Flags.** Any coach promising instant results (lose 20 pounds in 10 days!), requiring you to purchase a certain brand of products, refusing to provide client testimonials, or offering only generic programs should be avoided.

About Randall S. Hansen, Ph.D.

DR. RANDALL HANSEN is an educator, ethicist, advocate, and thought-leader for HEALING. Having been on a successful wellness journey that turned into a healing journey, all Dr. Hansen wants is to help other people find TRUE healing — not symptom management — because true healing opens us up to finally understanding who we are, what we are meant to do, and how to live a joy-filled life.

Websites: RandallShansen.com, TriumphOverTraumaBook.com, and HealMeWhole.com
LinkedIn: Linkedin.com/in/randallshansen
Instagram: @empoweringpines

CHAPTER 10:
How to Find a Forest/Nature Therapy Guide, from Kat Novotna, M.A.

Forest Therapy, Nature Therapy, Forest Bathing, or Shinrin-yoku. Several terms pointing to the same somatic-sensory practice where nature is the therapist and the guide opens the doors. The power of this nature-based well-being practice is in the deep reconnection between humans and the rest of nature.

It is a practice that will help rest your thinking mind, reset your nervous system, and allow nature to heal you on the physiological, mental, and emotional level — a truly holistic approach that no medical drug can guarantee without negative side effects!

Warning… Forest therapy can have powerful side effects (benefits): the deep affection for the planet, sense of belonging, well-being, and peace of mind that you rediscover may inspire you to do things you could never have imagined!

How to Find a Local Forest Therapy/Forest Bathing Guide

Guides may use different terms to describe their work. They might call themselves a Forest Therapy Guide, Forest Bathing Guide, Nature Therapy Guide, or Shinrin-yoku Guide, depending on the organization where they were trained as well as their personal preferences.

An important aspect that can inform you about a particular guide is to notice how they describe their work. The verbiage they use informs you about whether what they offer actually is forest bathing as opposed to other practices and modalities (like shamanic journeys, nature coaching, psychotherapy in nature, yoga or breathwork in nature, etc.).

While different guides can have slightly different approaches, these are some keywords to look for in descriptions of guided Forest Bathing experiences:

- Sensory immersion, using your senses to connect and be with nature
- Slowing down
- Invitational character of the activities offered (they are called invitations)
- Self-regulated experience
- Nature is the therapist, not the person or the guide
- Embodiment
- Relational aspect of the practice, reciprocity
- Radical hospitality & inclusion: everyone is welcome
- Non-prescriptive: there is no right or wrong way of doing Forest Bathing

Forest Bathing in its pure form is a culturally and spiritually neutral practice. While some people can have profound, even spiritual experiences, these should not be the reason to join, and it is not a Forest bathing guide's role to promise or facilitate them.

What Does a Typical Forest Bathing Experience Look Like?

A forest bathing experience will typically last about 2 – 3 hours. Shorter sessions are possible as a way to get to know the practice, but a full-length session is recommended. The gentle walks can take place in forests, city parks, or botanical gardens, but also on the beach or in smaller nature areas that are well-accessible for city inhabitants. They can be guided in person, or remotely with participants connecting online with the guide, group, and their local nature wherever they are.

A typical forest bathing experience will start with a short introduction of the guide, natural area, the practice, and some practicalities that are good to know for your safety and for everyone to feel welcome.

After the introduction, the guide will offer you a series of sensory-based invitations that can help you slow down, awaken your senses and body, and connect with nature, with a few moments of invitational sharing with the group throughout.

A typical forest bathing experience will end with a tea ceremony (in which the drink is produced from forest plants) that includes a few simple snacks that can be enjoyed together under the trees to slowly come back. Variations are possible, so please do not consider the above description as the only and right way of forest bathing!

What Makes a Good Forest Bathing Guide?

There are no good or bad guides — just different approaches. Some characteristics that might help you recognize a well-trained and experienced Forest Bathing guide:

- Certified by one of the official international or local training organizations.
- Experienced, actively guiding.
- Describing the practice in the above indicated or similar wordings.
- Connected to other guides, guide networks, or organizations.

Last but not least: The most accurate and trustworthy indicator that can help you find a good Forest Bathing guide is your own body. Join a guide for a walk and notice if you feel that their guiding embodies the nature connection, inner spaciousness, radical hospitality this practice represents. If the guide opens the doors for you so that you can slow down and reconnect, you have a good guide. If they keep you in your thinking mind or talking about your life situation and give you complicated exercises, you can probably look further.

About Kat Novotna, M.A.

KAT NOVOTNA, M.A., is a Forest Therapy Guide, founder of Eco-NIDRA™ and Way Back Home, Mentor in Presence & Self-Care, Kintsugi artist, and mom of one little Viking. Her passion and mission are to help people reconnect with nature, with themselves and with others. She has 20+ years of experience in training and community-building.

Websites: www.waybackhome.info and www.econidra.com
LinkedIn: www.linkedin.com/in/kat-novotna-723b71166
Instagram: @waybackhome_kat

CHAPTER 11:

How to Find a Psychedelic Guide/ Facilitator, from Randall Hansen, Ph.D.

Are you on a path to healing? Are you seeking an experienced guide or facilitator to assist you on an intentional psychedelic journey?

One of the biggest problems we face in the current marketplace is that all psychedelics are federally illegal, except for a few pockets of decriminalization in several states. In fact, only ketamine is available legally — through state-licensed clinics — across the U.S. (and around the world). But don't let the legal status stop you from exploring which of the medicines might be best for YOUR healing.

Thus, the big issue with psychedelics is two-fold: First, sourcing the medicine; second, finding a coach/guide.

Legally, I am not about to touch the first issue, but it is typically solved by finding a facilitator/guide — who can then lead you to sources to purchase the medicine. *Do not try and buy the medicine on your own!*

If it's your first psychedelic experience, it makes sense that you would want an experienced person to be there with you, to guide you and keep you out of harm's way. The mantra of most professional guides is all about harm reduction — constructing a safe environment for the psychedelic experience.

Thus, the key to the whole healing process is finding a psychedelic guide. Happily, because what these people do is perfectly legal (because they do not supply the medicine directly), many are out in the open and even have websites and social media profiles.

Let's take a closer look at these terms:

- **Tripsitter:** someone who is solely to hold space for you, making sure you are safe. These people can be trained, but could also be a sober partner, family member, or friend.
- **Guide/Facilitator:** someone who has experience working with other people in altered states and has often undergone certain trainings in working with psychedelics. Some may have advanced degrees, even be therapists.
- **Healer:** someone who claims they have been given natural healing talents and has dedicated their lives to fostering their healing abilities for the benefits of those who need healing.

Strategies for finding a guide/healer/facilitator:

1. **Word-of-mouth.** It's most likely at least someone you know is connected to the psychedelics movement. If not, consider joining one or more psychedelic societies and not only find your community (which is an ESSENTIAL part of the healing), but get referrals for facilitators/guides.
2. **Psychedelic portals.** These site often have detailed articles on tripsitting and often have links to various tripsitters and guides. You can even search LinkedIn for a psychedelic facilitator!
3. **Psychedelic guide companies.** Companies such as Psychedelic Passage do all the work for you in vetting facilitators, so all you need to decide is which medicine and which facilitator.

As you begin your research, you might want to make a list of criteria for evaluating potential guides, including:

- Level of training, education;
- Trauma, healing background;
- Continuing work on their own self-healing journey;
- Amount of personal experience with psychedelics;
- Number of ceremonies/journeys they have facilitated;
- Medicines they work with;
- Amount of coaching (pre and post) offered;
- Cost;
- Availability.

Final Thoughts: Do not work with a coach/guide who does not resonate with you, who is not doing the work on themselves, or whose ego/expertise seems overblown. Why? Read my article, Don't Make My Ayahuasca Mistake (http://www.empoweringadvice.com/ayahuasca.html). My partner and I also shared our experience on a podcast: https://www.youtube.com/watch?v=weCcNfDUWCY

About Randall S. Hansen, Ph.D.

DR. RANDALL HANSEN is an educator, ethicist, advocate, and thought-leader for HEALING. Having been on a successful wellness journey that turned into a healing journey, all Dr. Hansen wants is to help other people find TRUE healing — not symptom management — because true healing opens us up to finally understanding who we are, what we are meant to do, and how to live a joy-filled life.

Websites: RandallShansen.com, TriumphOverTraumaBook.com, and HealMeWhole.com
LinkedIn: Linkedin.com/in/randallshansen
Instagram: @empoweringpines

CHAPTER 12:
How to Find an Econidra Teacher, from Kat Novotna, M.A.

Econidra is a deeply relaxing, nature-based practice that helps people reconnect with nature and with themselves (their inner nature). It is a blend of Forest Bathing and the ancient practice of yoga Nidra – with healing effects for the physical, mental and emotional body. As a marriage of these two practices, it has elements and benefits of both worlds, offered in a very accessible way.

Some of the reported, recorded, and scientifically proven benefits of Econidra include:

- Lowered levels of stress hormones;
- Deep relaxation and feeling more energized;
- Improved sleep;
- Improved digestion and appetite regulation;
- Balanced blood pressure and blood glucose;
- Improved athletic performance;
- Pain relief;
- Improved mood, focus and creativity;
- Inspiration and improved ability to think out-of-the box;
- Sense of inner peace and improved relationships;
- Greater self-awareness and self-acceptance;
- Greater sense of connectedness with nature and other people.

What Does a Typical Econidra Session Look Like?

A typical Econidra session will last about 40 to 50 minutes. Shorter sessions are possible too, but not shorter than 15 to

20 minutes. The sessions are being offered outdoors in nature, indoors in yoga, meditation, and wellness centers, or remotely guided online where you can join from home.

A teacher will offer you a brief introduction and invite you to lie down on your back in the Shavasana pose or any other position that is comfortable for you. They will invite you to reduce any possible distractions, to cover yourself with a blanket, support your body with extra cushions if needed, and to adjust your audio volume if online.

Throughout the session, they will first guide you on a journey through your senses, then a pilgrimage through your body (also known as the rotation of consciousness), and finally, on a journey through the Earth guided by nature soundscapes. Their guidance will help your brain waves to slow down and your body to get into the parasympathetic nervous system dominance. They will help you get out of your thinking mind by first focusing on your senses, then withdrawing from your senses and shifting your awareness to the inner body.

Once you've entered the slow brain waves that will make you float between wakefulness and sleep, the guide will invite you to visualize any heart-felt wish you might have to plant a seed of positive change into this receptive state of consciousness. After the triple journey, they will skillfully guide you back, so that you can continue with your day, take a moment to reflect, or get to sleep.

How to Find an Econidra Teacher

To practice Econidra, you can find an Econidra teacher in your area by searching on the internet. You might find teachers offering sessions for the public close to where you live. Many

Econidra teachers also offer their sessions as a part of various kinds of well-being retreats and/or in combination with yoga, Forest Bathing, Reiki, sound healing, massage, and other healing and well-being modalities.

Some teachers specialize in offering Econidra sessions to various special groups and populations, for example, people suffering from long Covid, cancer patients, those in addiction recovery, teenagers with special needs, pregnant women, women going through menopause, people processing grief, those who wish to strengthen their connection with their pets, and so much more.

As an alternative to in-person sessions offered indoors or outdoors in nature, you can also join a remotely guided session offered online, or get a recorded session guided by one of the certified teachers.

The following tips might be helpful:

- Look for a trained and certified teacher, they will call themselves a Certified EcoNIDRA Teacher, or alternatively a Certified EcoNIDRA Guide.
- Apart from deep relaxation, nature should definitely play a role. Econidra teachers and participants partner with nature for every session and part of each session is also an Earth journey with nature sounds.
- Econidra as a practice and the Econidra language are culturally and spiritually neutral. While participants can have profound experiences during and after the sessions and these become part of their authentic experience, Econidra teachers should not advertise, promise, or try to facilitate any spiritual experiences. Deep relaxation and reconnecting with nature and oneself are at the core of the practice.

- Before you join a program or retreat, it might be helpful to hear an Econidra teacher's voice to see if their voice color, pace, and way of speaking resonate with you. It might be a good idea to contact a teacher to ask if they offer single sessions or if you can purchase a recorded session before you join a larger program.

About Kat Novotna, M.A.

KAT NOVOTNA, M.A., is a Forest Therapy Guide, founder of Eco-NIDRA™ and Way Back Home, Mentor in Presence & Self-Care, Kintsugi artist, and mom of one little Viking. Her passion and mission are to help people reconnect with nature, with themselves and with others. She has 20+ years of experience in training and community-building.

Websites: www.waybackhome.info and www.econidra.com
LinkedIn: www.linkedin.com/in/kat-novotna-723b71166
Instagram: @waybackhome_kat

CHAPTER 13:
How to Find a Somatic Healer/ Therapist, from Dr. Michael Hofrath

Somatic psychology or body psychotherapy moves beyond talk therapy to include an individual's lived experience and bodily-felt sense, as a primary means of understanding the unconscious processes that dictate our conscious thoughts, behavior, and actions.

Somatic psychotherapy is an integrated treatment of the body, mind, and soul viewed as a functional whole. Somatic psychotherapists assist clients in exploring the subtle nuances revealed by soma (the body). Somatic therapists are trained to listen actively and observe the subtle shifts in the body most people aren't aware of.

For example, deep or shallow breathing, the amount of tension held in the body, and the level of tension in different areas of the body all provide valuable information for the somatic therapist. Somatic healers will observe how grounded a client is in their body, be aware if the client is present in the moment, living in the stories of the past, or worrying about the future. Eye contact (and the lack thereof) and bodily movements are all extremely informative features.

Somatic healers will use breathwork, mindfulness techniques, movement exercises, and even touch to assist clients in exploring their feelings and bodily sensations. A client's posture, gestures, and various other expressions also provide vital information to a somatic healer.

When looking for a somatic healer, it's important to consider several qualities and skills that can contribute to a positive therapeutic experience. Here are some key factors to consider:

1. **Training and Qualifications:** Ensure that the therapist has received appropriate training and holds relevant qualifications in somatic therapy or a related field. Look for certifications, licenses, or memberships in professional organizations.

2. **Experience:** Consider the therapist's experience working with clients who have similar concerns or goals as you. Ask about their experience in somatic therapy and any specialized training or areas of expertise they have.

3. **Empathy and Compassion:** A somatic therapist should possess empathy, compassion, and the ability to create a safe and non-judgmental space for you to explore and express your emotions and experiences. This quality helps establish a trusting therapeutic relationship.

4. **Effective Communication:** Look for a therapist who communicates clearly, listens attentively, and is responsive to your needs and concerns. A good somatic therapist should be able to explain concepts, techniques, and processes in a way that you can understand.

5. **Sensitivity to Body and Non-Verbal Cues:** Somatic therapy focuses on the connection between the mind and body. A skilled somatic therapist should be attuned to non-verbal cues, body language, and subtle shifts in your physical sensations or expressions. They should be able to guide you in exploring and understanding the wisdom of your body.

6. **Boundaries and Ethics:** Ensure that the therapist maintains professional boundaries and adheres to ethical guidelines. This includes maintaining confidentiality, respecting your autonomy, and providing a safe and secure therapeutic environment.
7. **Collaboration and Partnership:** A good somatic therapist should view therapy as a collaborative process and work in partnership with you. They should involve you in setting goals, exploring treatment options, and adapting the therapeutic approach to your individual needs and preferences.
8. **Continued Professional Development:** Look for a therapist who engages in ongoing professional development, stays updated with the latest research and advancements in somatic therapy, and demonstrates a commitment to their own growth and learning.
9. **Trust and Intuition:** Ultimately, trust your intuition and assess how comfortable and safe you feel with the therapist. Trust and a positive therapeutic relationship are crucial for the effectiveness of somatic therapy.

Final Thoughts: It can be helpful to schedule an initial consultation or interview with potential somatic therapists to get a sense of their approach, to ask questions, and to determine if they are the right fit for you. Remember, finding the right therapist is a personal process, and it's important to choose someone with whom you feel comfortable and supported on your healing journey.

About Dr. Michael Hofrath

DR. MICHAEL HOFRATH offers a somatic, transpersonal, and shamanic approach to assist clients in moving through adverse conditioned behavior, old programming, limiting belief patterns, ancestral trauma and cellular repatterning for movement into alignment with one's authentic self. Additionally, he works with psycho-spiritual crisis resolution, dream tending, mandala-art therapy, experiential (outdoor) healing modalities, Hero's Journey rite of passage initiations, and psychedelic-assisted therapies and integration.

Website: https://bodymindwholeness.com/

CHAPTER 14:
How to Find a Sound Healer, from Bree Dellerson, L.Ac.

Not everyone who has the tools knows how to wield them.

A sound healer is a guide who takes you on a vibrational journey. Sound healers are not just playing their gongs or bowls. They are in tune with themselves, their instruments, and the people for whom they're playing.

It is a sonic dialogue that happens on multidimensional levels between the practitioner and the client(s). There is a deep listening to the music the client emanates and a compassionate response with the sound needed to create coherence, alignment, and balance.

Sound is medicine. Sound healing addresses health on all levels of being... through space and time. It penetrates the body-mind. Like water, it flows through the aspects of self the mind struggles to reach.

Sound touches tender places from this lifetime and others, unearthing emotions that had been lying deep beneath the surface. *The sound transforms pain.* It restores movement of your vital Life Force and with it, health.

There is much science and research to support what the ancients have known around the power of sound healing. In modern terms, it entrains the brainwaves to healing and meditative states, stimulates the vagus nerve, boosts the immune system, benefits the heart and circulation, activates the meridians and our DNA, and more. Other benefits can include mood enhancement, pain reduction, increased productivity, and better sleep.

On the emotional and spiritual level, it has a profound effect on our consciousness and can help transform and clear stuck emotions and trauma stored in the body-mind.

Quality not quantity. It's not about how many bowls or gongs or tuning forks a sound healer possesses. *It's how skillfully they use the tools they do have to bring you to state of healing.*

Strategies for Finding a Sound Healer

1. **Word of mouth.** This is always the best reference. Once you start looking, you'll draw the right people to you at the right time.
2. **Explore the sound schools in person and online.** Many have open house events, classes you can audit and experience gifted teachers and pioneers in the field. I was blessed to study with David Gibson, Steven Halpern, and Randy Masters, to name just a few.
3. **Visit your local yoga studios.** Many yoga studios host kirtans and sound healing events. (Some massage/body therapists do so as well.)
4. **Social Media.** YouTube is a wonderful place to find people. You can search by the instrument you love and see what comes up. I've found a handpan musician I love who also teaches you how to play... something I've been considering exploring for my own medicine.
5. **Voice.** Sound healing is not just about the bowls, there are many ways sound is used in healing. Chanting and toning are two powerful sound healing modalities. Your voice is a transformative healing tool that you have available at all

times. Kirtans are wonderful ways to experience the power of chanting in person.

6. **Training.** I am a believer in education. Do they have to be certified to be masterful? No. But having experienced and studied Sound Healing with many different practitioners since 1997, training can help deepen their connection to their craft and expand their intuitive ability.

Final Note: How Do You Know if The Sounder Healer You Discovered is Good?

You'll feel it. It's that simple. Your body will know.

I've had to leave certain sound baths because I was agitated after 15 minutes. I've also achieved complete bliss where everything turned to white light. *Trust your body.*

Not every practitioner is right for every person. Find the one who is right for you.

*One of several studies showcasing the healing benefits from sound: https://doi.org/10.1177/2156587216668109

About Bree Dellerson, L.Ac.

Bree is a Licensed Acupuncturist, sound healer, and clairvoyant who has been helping people for more than 22 years attain vibrational health by awakening the healing intelligence of their bodymind. Her unique skill set helps her quickly and accurately identify the dissonance in one's field while simultaneously restoring harmony and flow of their vital life force.

Website: BreeDellersonLAc.com
Email: bree@breedellersonlac.com

CHAPTER 15:
How to Find a Certified EMDR Therapist, from Christopher Brown, LICSW

About EMDR

EMDR is short for eye-movement desensitization and reprocessing. Acknowledged by institutions like the U.S. Department of Veterans Affairs and the World Health Organization, EMDR is a top-tier treatment method for helping individuals heal from the psychological impacts of trauma.

Developed by Francine Shapiro in the early 1990s, EMDR utilizes bilateral stimulation to help the brain process the cognitive, emotional, and physical impacts of a traumatic memory or stressor. Over the years, EMDR has been studied in a wide range of contexts and proven highly effective as a treatment option for PTSD and other trauma-related mental health conditions.

Research has shown the bilateral stimulation involved in EMDR does two things in the brain simultaneously: 1) activates the hippocampus, the brain region responsible for vivid memory recall linked to emotion and 2) suppresses the amygdala, the brain region responsible for the fight or flight response. The result is EMDR puts the brain in a state that is ripe for efficient processing and ultimately, healing.

How Does EMDR Work?

One way to think of how EMDR works is to imagine a cluttered closet (trauma), bursting at the hinges, overwhelming you every time you walk by or try to open it to get something inside. With the help of a therapist guiding you through the EMDR process, you can go through everything in the closet, clearing out that which no longer serves you, keeping that which does, and making space for new things to exist.

Now the closet is clean, tidy, and you feel a sense of relief when you look inside. It's important to note EMDR does not make the closet disappear, rather, it helps change your *relationship* with the closet (or the trauma) and allows you to integrate it into your life in a way that is healthy and productive.

What to Expect

When you work with an EMDR therapist, you can expect a few sessions focused on preparation, learning more about you and your traumas, teaching you a few skills you can use if you experience emotional distress, and developing a plan for how to approach the trauma work.

Once you have identified a target to start with, you move into using the bilateral stimulation component of EMDR to process trauma. This can be done in various ways, including eyes following a therapist's fingers, a dot on a screen, or a light bar. Or it may involve holding alternating vibrating tappers in your palms, or performing your own taps on your knees or shoulders, matching the pace of the therapist. You will experience this bilateral stimulation while focusing on the specific trauma and noticing the corresponding thoughts, images, emotions, and physical sensations that come up. The therapist will guide you through this process in a contained way and most sessions last from 1-2 hours.

Depending on the complexity of your experience, you may spend a few sessions focused on one traumatic experience, or you may spend several sessions clearing the emotional burden around many different experiences. It is common for individuals to complete several EMDR sessions before they fully experience the relief they are looking for.

Certified EMDR Therapists

EMDR is an advanced technique that should only be performed by trained professionals. Attempting EMDR on your own or with someone who has not completed advanced training and consultation can lead to less than desired results, or in some cases, severe harm. While seeking an EMDR therapist, be sure to ask about their level of experience and training.

Working with a Certified EMDR Therapist who has been certified by the EMDR International Association (EMDRIA), you will be working with a therapist who has completed not just advanced training, but also more than 20 hours of consultation with an Approved Consultant to verify they are following best practices for EMDR.

How to Find a Certified EMDR Therapist

You can find EMDRIA Certified EMDR Therapists by using the therapist directory found on the EMDRIA website: https://www.emdria.org/find-an-emdr-therapist/

About Christopher Brown, LICSW

Christopher Brown, LICSW has more than 8 years of experience as an EMDR provider and consults with other professionals who are pursuing EMDR certification and training. He is a Certified EMDR Therapist with EMDRIA. As founder and owner of Peak Psychotherapy, PLLC, Chris uses EMDR and Psychedelic Integration to help clients achieve their goals, while empowering other therapists to do the same.

Website: www.peakpsychotherapy.co/

CHAPTER 16:

How to Find a Reiki Master/Intuitive Energy Healer, from Angela Lerro

To heal is to become whole and often we frantically seek external sources to try to find the answers to what's causing our illnesses, but not so often do we dive inward to address the connection between our disease and our mind, body, and spirit.

While understanding the physical root cause is helpful in terms of diagnosis, there is always an emotional and metaphysical energetic component to what made us get sick in the first place. Many people underestimate the power that our stored trauma and negative emotions have in playing in our health, but after years and years of not being addressed, they can eventually wreak havoc on our nervous system.

When our nervous system becomes dysregulated, our body's immune system also becomes dysregulated—as the two go hand in hand. The word "emotion" means energy in motion, and that is the sole purpose of what Reiki is. Reiki is a Japanese healing technique that promotes stress reduction and relaxation so the body can come back into balance and heal itself naturally.

The benefits of Reiki:

- Fosters relaxation
- Reduces anxiety
- Lowers blood pressure
- Releases trauma and unwanted emotions
- Decreases pain
- Increases vitality

- Promotes better sleep
- Aids with digestion
- Reduces brain fog and increases mental clarity
- Grounding
- Increases intuition and connection to Source Energy

Since we all are uniquely composed of different energy, not every practitioner is going to connect or resonate... so finding the right healer that you feel is a good fit for you is especially important.

Reiki and energy healing is a very sacred and intimate practice so you want to be mindful of who is connecting with your energy.

When searching for the right Reiki Healer, I have found the following to be the most helpful.

1. **Ask people you know and trust first.** Hearing personal stories and examples of how a particular practitioner works will help you decide if their style resonates most with you. Refrain from using Yelp or Google reviews, as they are not always authentic.
2. **Find an interactive social media group,** such as on Facebook, and create a post asking if anyone had any experiences working with a Reiki Master and/or if they had anyone that they would personally recommend.
3. **Connect with local yoga studios, crystal/spiritual shops, and wellness centers;** these places are most often connected with Reiki Practitioners and/or the owners are practitioners themselves.
4. **Look at social media accounts under hashtags like #reiki #reikihealer on Instagram.** See if/how they live is in alignment with your healing goals. Read about their healing story or journey and see how you feel. Is it authentic? Do

you resonate? Do you feel hopeful?

5. **Make a list of intentions of what you are trying to accomplish and ask questions:**
   - What level of training do they have?
   - Do they have any areas of expertise: trauma, chronic illness, autoimmune, etc.?
   - How long of a commitment are they asking for?
   - Cost?
   - What can you expect after a session?
   - What is their expectation of you?
   - Do you have to be in person or do they work remotely?
   - Are there any side effects?

Final Note: Be patient with your healing and give yourself time. It is a marathon, not a sprint. Remember you didn't get sick overnight so you can't heal overnight. Addressing the mind, body, and soul together is essential to achieving full wellness and healing.

About Angela Lerro

Angela Lerro is an Intuitive Reiki Master, Clairvoyant Medium since childhood and Holistic Health, and Wellness Practitioner. After battling breast cancer at a young age and chronic Lyme Disease for the last several years, Angela has healed herself and has made it her mission to combine her intuitive gifts with the knowledge and wisdom she has gained so that she can turn her pain into purpose. Angela has had her Holistic Healing Practice for almost ten years and works remotely with clients all over the world. You can learn more about her work via LinkedIn or on Instagram... please feel free to send her a message.

Instagram: @Anglerro28 or @Meatbasedmedium
LinkedIn: www.linkedin.com/in/angela-lerro-28b7bb9b/

CHAPTER 17:
How To Find A Microdosing Coach, from Matt Simpson

Are you curious about all the buzz centered around microdosing psychedelics? Are you seeking an experienced guide to help you safely navigate this emerging frontier?

Finding a microdosing coach involves several steps to ensure you connect with a knowledgeable and trustworthy individual. Microdosing involves taking small amounts of substances like psychedelics (e.g., LSD or psilocybin) in sub-perceptual doses to potentially achieve spiritual, cognitive, or emotional benefits.

There is a wondrous opportunity with this misunderstood strategy for healing and deepening into self-love: clarity and connection... so finding the right guide is *imperative*.

Here's how you might find a microdosing coach:

- **Research:** Begin by researching the concept of microdosing and understanding its potential benefits and risks. This will help you make informed decisions and ask the right questions when looking for a coach.
- **Legality:** Make sure to understand the legal status of microdosing substances in your country or state. There is a decriminalization movement happening across the U.S., but these substances are still illegal at the federal level, so proceed with caution.
- **Online Search:** Look for microdosing coaches online through search engines, social media, and relevant online forums

or Meetup communities. Websites, blogs, and social media profiles dedicated to psychedelic integration might provide leads.

- **Check Credentials and Experience:** When identifying potential coaches, check their credentials and experience. Look for any pertinent certifications, training, or relevant qualifications: Have they written a book? Do they have a podcast?
- **Reviews and Testimonials:** Look for reviews or testimonials from previous clients. Positive feedback can give you an idea of their coaching style, effectiveness, and professionalism.
- **Initial Consultation:** Contact potential coaches and schedule an initial consultation. This can be a phone call or video chat where you can discuss your goals concerns, and ask any questions you might have. Pay attention to how comfortable you feel during this conversation and whether the coach seems knowledgeable and empathetic.
- **Ethics and Approach:** Inquire about the coach's ethical approach to microdosing and psychedelic experiences. They should prioritize safety, legality, and responsible use. Ask about their coaching methods and how they tailor their approach to individual needs. Microdosing often inspires healthy habits, so a comprehensive understanding of holistic health is a huge bonus.
- **Cost and Commitment:** Discuss the cost of coaching sessions and any potential packages they offer. Make sure you are comfortable with the financial commitment before proceeding.
- **Compatibility:** A good coach-client relationship is crucial. Please ensure you feel comfortable, understood, and respected by the coach. Mutual trust and rapport are

essential for effective coaching. Please inquire about the challenges they have overcome to live an integrated life.

- **Customization:** A reputable coach will tailor their guidance to your needs and goals. Beware of dogmatic rigidity; they should be open to adjusting their approach based on your feedback and experiences.
- **Legal and Medical Considerations:** A responsible coach will discuss legal and medical considerations with you. They should advise you on potential risks and interactions and encourage you to consult with a medical professional before starting any microdosing regimen, especially when tapering off of medications.
- **Continued Support:** Microdosing can be an ongoing process, so inquire about the coach's availability for continued support. Check whether they offer follow-up sessions or ongoing guidance. Does the practitioner have experience with higher doses and a firm understanding of the supreme importance of integration?

Final Thoughts: Remember that microdosing is a new cultural phenomenon. Be wary of untrained professionals offering professional services. Trust is the most crucial factor when choosing a guide to help you work with these Sacred medicines.

Take your time to find a coach who aligns with your values, prioritizes safety, and has the necessary expertise to guide you responsibly.

About Matt Simpson

Matt Simpson is a Microdose Mentor, guiding disenchanted high-achievers back to the path of passion and possibility. His 1-on-1 Worthy Fight Empowerment Coaching is all about demystifying psychedelics, igniting hope, and fast-tracking personal growth. He is also author of the powerful book, Worth the Fight: A Guide to Spirituality, Psychedelic Medicines, and Overcoming Trauma.

Meetup: www.meetup.com/psychedelics-and-limitless-personal-growth/
Website: www.worththefightbook.org
Email: matt@nltrans.org

CHAPTER 18:
How to Find an Ecotherapist, from Lizabeth Kashinsky

Ecopsychology, born out of the environmental movement, was formally named and defined as a field of study in 1992. Ecopsychology recognizes that the perceived separation between humans and the rest of nature is at the root of many environmental, health, and social issues today.

Ecopsychology arose from inherent connections humans have with the Earth, and many aspects of ecotherapy have indigenous and ancient roots. Ecopsychology recognizes that humans are a part of nature, and that our health and well-being are deeply intertwined with the health and well-being of the Earth.

Ecotherapy, considered applied ecopsychology, is an umbrella term for varied forms of therapies and practices that draw upon the healing effects of nature connection, ranging from improving healing in hospitals by incorporating garden settings, wilderness rites of passage programs, forest bathing and other sensory awareness practices, ecoart therapy, animal-assisted therapy, restoration work, horticulture therapy, bearing witness and offering ritual to wounded places, and ecosomatic therapy.

Ecotherapy is also offered by some licensed mental health providers who might bring elements of nature connection practices into a clinical setting (also called ecopsychotherapy). Clinical ecotherapy can be done indoors or outdoors (e.g., walk and talk therapy).

Another important aspect of ecotherapy that is becoming more well known is the recognition of environmental grief, eco-anxiety, eco-despair, ecological grief, and other terms used to describe the mental health impacts due to the loss of the natural world and climate change challenges we face as a global community. Mental health professionals, ecopsychologists, and coaches can support individuals in coping with these types of challenges.

How to Find an Ecotherapist

Finding an ecotherapist depends on your personal needs. Ecotherapists are as varied as there are types of ecotherapy. Some licensed mental health practitioners offer ecotherapy sessions as a part of their mental health therapy and sessions may be covered by insurance.

Ecotherapists may hold a degree in ecopsychology, but not all are licensed mental health workers. While not a comprehensive list, you may also find an ecotherapy provider through outdoor educators, life coaches, wilderness rites of passage guides, horticulturists, somatic therapists and body workers — if they have a nature connection component — or animal-assisted therapy professionals.

An important consideration when seeking an ecotherapist is the language used to describe their work. Level one ecotherapists may only value the healing benefits to humans and might use terms such as "using nature to heal," whereas level two ecotherapists recognize reciprocity between humans and the rest of nature, due to the interconnectedness between humans and the Earth.

What Makes a Good Ecotherapist?

Characteristics that might help you recognize a well-trained and experienced ecotherapist:

- Has experiences demonstrating their own deep relationship with the natural world, and/or through trainings/certifications depending on their field of expertise;
- Recognizes interconnectedness and reciprocity;
- Offers embodiment and sensory awareness practices;
- Offers mindfulness practices in nature;
- Is trauma-informed and recognizes that trauma is not exclusive to the human experience (e.g., not causing trauma to animals in equine therapy programs);
- Has a willingness to share and answer questions you might have before using their services. Many ecotherapists may offer a free 15-minute or longer consultation so you can determine whether they meet your needs;
- Can demonstrate an understanding of the difference between level 1 or level 2 ecotherapy;
- Doing their work with cultural sensitivity by honoring and respecting indigenous cultures and practices; does not participate in cultural appropriation;
- Has a good understanding of, and acknowledgement of, the history of the land and indigenous peoples of the places where they live and work;
- Are inclusive: all beings are recognized as having equal value, whether human or nonhuman;
- Embraces diversity and has a social justice component to their work, focusing on decolonizing, as colonization has contributed to the Western cultural disconnect from nature;

- Invitational; does not support forcing (e.g., animal assisted therapy animals are able to choose and are not forced into situations that may be detrimental to their well-being).

Final Thoughts: Ecotherapy is accessible to each of us at any time, and we do not necessarily need a guide, nor do we need access to wild nature or wilderness.

Connecting with the natural world can be as simple as cultivating a relationship with a tree in our yard or neighborhood, a special place in nature that we can visit regularly to connect... or even something as simple as a single house plant or stone. Ecotherapy invites us to stay open, pay attention, and to be present with the world around us.

About Lizabeth Kashinsky

Lizabeth Kashinsky, M.A., holds a master's degree in Transpersonal psychology with an emphasis in ecopsychology, is a 500-hour RYT, and a certified ecotherapist. Her passion is to connect others to nature and she holds workshops, retreats, and classes in Hawaii. She is also passionate about healing with horses.

Website: www.nature-connects.com
LinkedIn: www.linkedin.com/in/lizabeth-kashinsky-14429930/
Instagram: @nature_connectshi

CHAPTER 19:

How to Find a Breathwork Practitioner, from Marissa Kosolofski

Breathwork is a versatile and accessible tool for gaining physical, mental, emotional, and spiritual well-being. Nailing down specific benefits and experiences can be tricky as they vary greatly depending on technique used and the practitioner's intention. Getting clear on your personal goals and objectives for your practice is a great place to start.

Just like *Fitness* and *Yoga, Breathwork* is an umbrella term that includes various styles, techniques, and methodologies in which the practitioner takes breath in and breathes it back out. Depending on your breath of choice, breathwork can fall into two categories:

- **Breath Awareness** — a practice where you simply observe the natural breath as it is;
- **Conscious Breath** — the breath is controlled into deliberate patterns, moving the breather in and out of states of calm or excitement.

Knowing your breathwork goals is an important place to start. Here are some common intentions people have when beginning their breathwork journey:

- **Stress Reduction** — specific breathing techniques can regulate the body's nervous system by activating the relaxation.
- **Emotional Regulation** — some breath control techniques help folks to skillfully respond to emotional triggers by fostering mindfulness and presence.

- **Physical Health** — Breathwork techniques, like diaphragmatic breathing, have been shown to enhance lung function, improve cardiovascular health, and boost overall vitality.
- **Pain Management** — the breather's ability to reduce bodily tension and promote muscle relaxation is beneficial for folks experiencing physical discomfort from muscle tightness. The breath is also a valuable tool for folks dealing with chronic pain.
- **Mental Focus** — Playing with the oxygen levels in the body can improve mental clarity, concentration and focus which is beneficial for productivity and cognitive performance.
- **Self-Awareness** — Breathwork often involves paying close attention to the breath and the sensations in the body, leading to greater self-awareness and a deeper understanding of one's thoughts, emotions, and physical sensations.
- **Creativity** — The breath can offer access to deeper levels of creativity and inspiration that are hard to reach with a busy inner critic.
- **Spiritual Exploration** — Breathwork is a beautiful vehicle to access expanded states of consciousness, creating a perception that goes beyond the ordinary, everyday level of consciousness.

Once you have determined your goals, you can look to understand how much you can accomplish on your own and where you might need additional support. You can find breath being facilitated online and in-person, at studios, retreats, and in the comfort of your own home in both individual and group settings.

Finding a reputable guide that you feel comfortable with will take some discovery. Some resources to find breathwork guides are:

- **Word-of-mouth** — Ask people in your community, especially in wellness and holistic communities; it should not be long before you find some names from trusted resources.
- **Online** — Try searching online or using your favorite social media platform. You should be able to find facilitators who are in your desired location and specialize in the style of breath that is aligned with your goals. Additionally, following them on social media can give you a perspective of their personality and up-to-date offerings.
- **Studios/Retreats** — Using a breathwork guide who already works for a studio or retreat is another great option, as the company has typically done the vetting for you.

Once you have found some options, it will be your responsibility to ensure your own quality control for a safe and effective experience. Considerations to keep in mind during your vetting process are:

- **Credentials & Training** — Confirm certification, years of experience, and continuing education/training in specific breathwork modalities or within related fields such as meditation, yoga, or counseling.
- **Ethical considerations** — Creating a safe and supportive environment is crucial, so ensure your facilitator understands boundaries and can maintain confidentiality by asking them about their code of conduct.
- **Safety protocols** — Breathwork comes with contraindications, so ask your guide about precautions related to breathwork especially if you have underlying health concerns. Every

facilitator should have protocols in place in the event of a possible adverse reaction.

- **Reviews & Testimonials** — Online is a great resource for reviews, but make sure you approach it with a neutral mind. Positive reviews are a great way to ensure effectiveness, but be sure to pay attention to any negative feedback and consider discussing any concerns you may have with your guide.
- **Time and money** — If the cost is outside your price range and located somewhere inconvenient, you probably will find yourself with too much tension to make the change into a lifestyle habit. Set yourself up for success with an accessible practitioner and style that still delivers against your goals.
- **Intuition** — There's something to be said about your gut instinct. If it doesn't feel right, consider this your permission to explore other options. Don't ever put yourself in a position where you don't feel safe with the guide's qualifications or approach.

Final Advice: Finding your style of breathwork and favorite breathwork guide will be an adventure. It might take some time to create your practice so please above all, be patient and remain curious.

Your breath is unique to you, just like your healing journey... so keep showing up, breath after breath.

About Marissa Kosolofski

Marissa Kosolofski is a psychedelic advocate, community builder, and the creatrix of The Golden Thread Studio, an online wellness studio specializing in breathwork journeys and self-care practices. Her mission to create connection such that people are present to the beauty of the human experience and the magic of everyday moments, was born from her own psychedelic-assisted transformation.

Website: www.thegoldenthreadstudio.com
Email: marissa@thegoldenthreadstudio.com
Instagram: @the_golden_thread_studio
LinkedIn: www.linkedin.com/in/marissakosolofski/

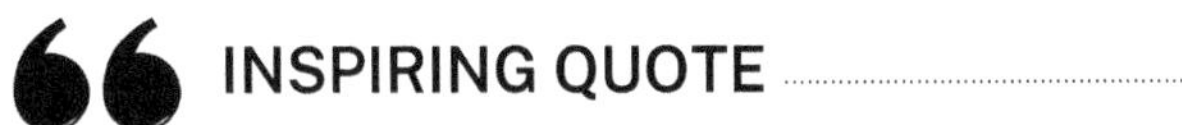

“Healing may not be so much about getting better, as about letting go of everything that isn't you — all of the expectations, all of the beliefs — and becoming who you are.” — Rachel Naomi Remen

PART THREE:
HEALING STORIES

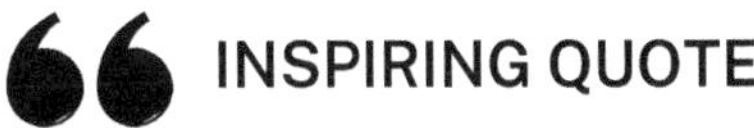

“I've experienced several different healing methodologies over the years — counseling, self-help seminars, and I've read a lot — but none of them will work unless you really want to heal.” — Lindsay Wagner

AUTHOR INSIGHT

I share my story among many others in the following pages, but your focus should be on finding one or more stories that resonate with you — and from which you can gain insights and a path for your own healing.

CHAPTER 20:
Healing Journey Story #1

Nature, Meditation, Love, and Mindfulness Healed Me

First Name: Ran

Age: Baby Boomer

Gender: Male

How/Why You Started on Healing Journey: My life was unraveling and I had lost my center.

Words That Describe Where You are in Your Healing Journey: Healed... and now want to help everyone else heal!

Most Valuable Thing You've Learned on Your Healing Journey: There's joy, beauty, and freedom from healing. You don't need to live in pain or in hiding.

Progress on Your Healing Journey: Done with the big stuff; the heavy lifting. Now it's about fine-tuning.

Hardest Part of Your Healing Journey: Doubting myself, doubting my spirituality, self-loathing.

Best Advice to Someone Just Starting Their Healing Journey: Please just start. It may take several steps and missteps and hurdles, but doing the work gets you the reward of true and complete healing.

My Healing Story:

My trauma story is trivial, especially compared to the trauma others have experienced. Yes, I know the rule of not comparing myself to others, but I state this here because a lot of people think the trauma they have experienced is trivial or not important — and that's simply not the case.

Trauma is trauma. Yes, there are some pretty horrible traumas people have endured, but as we dig deeper into our knowledge of trauma, we see that we ALL experience some form(s) of trauma.

This book discusses several healing modalities; research, try, and find the modalities that work best for you.

So, let me share my story.

Background

I grew up in an upper-middle-class, affluent neighborhood that was part of a working-class township. My dad was an organic chemist and my mom was a homemaker. Why they chose to live in that community — Short Hills, NJ, for anyone who knows it — I don't know. About half of all the fights/arguments my folks had was over money — the lack of it.

I wish I could ask my folks, now both deceased, why they chose to live there. We barely had enough to keep up with appearances, and as the youngest, I got all the second-hand stuff from my brothers and cousins. While neighbors had Range Rovers and Jaguars, we had a used, beat-up Chevy Impala.

As the youngest of four boys, I often felt invisible as a kid. My dad ruled the roost, and that roost was ruled by logic, fear, and the belt. No feelings allowed, at least none that would ever win an argument. My dad's temper was one to avoid at ALL costs. For the majority of my childhood, my dad was also a functioning alcoholic whose rage only seemed to emerge in the evenings.

I can't tell you how many times I got whipped (whether I deserved it or not), but I cleverly found a system of shoving magazines down my pants and he was usually too drunk to notice he was whacking paper and not me.

Then there were the times when he showed up drunk at my Boy Scout meetings when I was 12 or so. Oh, the joy of having a drunk father arguing with my Scoutmaster and other parents. Needless to say, I quit Scouts and any other evening activities that would involve needing a parent. I was less scared of the drunk driving than I was of the embarrassment.

Outwardly, we lived a nice life. My folks traveled some when my dad won awards or presented a paper at an academic conference. We did some traveling as a family, but it was pretty limited. My dad and I even went to a few NY Mets games, as I was the only son interested in sports.

My brothers are all quite different from me, and also as the youngest, I spent a lot of time amusing myself… in my younger days, I had an imaginary friend. Later, I climbed trees, rode my bike all over the place, and built a fort in the backyard (as a safe hiding place).

Home life was so bad that only my oldest brother ever invited anyone over… and I loved weekends when I could crash at a friend's house. I never had a "friends/schoolmates" birthday party and rarely attended other parties.

Luckily, I had my mom. She was my emotional center… and I think some of my trauma actually comes from the empathy I had for my mom when my dad screamed at her, called her names, and flaunted his *Playboy* magazines in front of her.

When I was around 7 or 8, I had a concussion (and TBI before they knew what that was) from a crazy bicycling accident where

I fell over my handlebars face-first into the pavement. I did go to the emergency room for stitches, but don't remember any other treatment.

When I was a teen and got my growth spurt, I became the peacemaker in my family, stepping in between my dad and anyone else... I just wanted peace and quiet.

I was always involved in our local Episcopal Church and loved being in a community that allowed me to be me and also serve my God.

Ironically, years later, I was sexually propositioned/assaulted by an Episcopal priest. Sadly, sexual abuse is rampant in our culture, and certainly in our so-called Christian culture.

I married pretty young, at age 24, thinking I was in love, but really just rescuing a friend who had gotten pregnant by another man. I raised that child and we had one of our own. Even though I was committed to the marriage, I soon discovered there was no real passion or true love in it, which led to many issues down the line. (Probably should have ended the marriage then, but we made the classic bad decision of staying together for the kids.)

To me, my biggest trauma was the night I knew my son was going to commit suicide. I was on my way to the emergency room after he had mutilated himself (I stayed home to clean up all the blood), when I got a call that he had escaped the hospital. I can vividly — to this day — see myself in my little red pickup truck sitting at a red light wondering what to do next... and steeling my heart in preparation for the news that he had accomplished his goal. I pushed the pain and hurt down and "compartmentalized" it in my heart.

My son lived that night, but my heart was not the same for almost two decades. I thought I had protected my heart, but really, it was *shattered*.

I gave up on the marriage, and sought a divorce half-heartedly. I acted out. Went out and got drunk with some of my students on too many nights. Watched a lot of porn. Contemplated multiple affairs... anything to show I was really still alive. I kind of liked living on the edge, waiting for the shit to hit the fan, but luckily never went down the cliched rabbit hole of sleeping with any students.

I started wearing masks (or fake personas) in every part of my life, hiding the brokenness within, which allowed me to "fit in" with whatever crowd I was interacting with — neighbors, colleagues, students, family, businesses, friends. With juggling all those masks, I was able to simply lose myself in those other personas. Truly, those masks were a survival mechanism, with me hanging by a thread.

I began to hate everything and everyone — so not like me. (My theme song for many, many years has been James Taylor's *You've Got a Friend.*)

Even with the hurt, self-hate, and uncontrolled trauma responses, I never once thought of going on any medications... other than St. John's Wort, which I tried, but did nothing for me. I did think often about getting in my truck and just disappearing, driving off to wherever; other times, I envisioned driving away, but instead of disappearing, driving the truck into an overpass concrete embankment to end things.

The Healing Begins

I suppose the first healing attempt started with couples therapy in an effort to save the marriage; the problem was less to do with the marriage and more to do with me. The counseling failed.

Call it God (though at the time I felt God had abandoned me), but somehow I decided the best thing for me was to move thousands of miles for a fresh start. It took a few months of searching, but I found 40 acres of forestland in desperate need of healing; ironic looking back, yes.

I spent the next 7 years or so basically alone in nature, in my forest, cutting down diseased trees, removing invasive species, and loving my days. I had lost faith in God, but found Divinity in the forest, with the trees and animals. I prayed or meditated daily... in the forest. I soon called my time in the forest as my time in nature's cathedral. *I experienced forest therapy without even knowing it.*

Those years in the forest, when I had that much time to myself, with myself, I found healing. I emerged from that time — when I had brought the entire 40 acres to good standing and health — as a new man... as my true self for the first time in perhaps 30 years... maybe for the *first time since I was a kid.*

I didn't really know much about trauma at that point, but I instinctively knew what was best for me... and the forest therapy was gold for me. I should note at the same time, I was also deep into my wellness regimen of healthy eating, exercise, and rebuilding self-love and self-respect.

Toward the end of my work (on myself and the forest), I knew I must be healing, because I started venturing out. I actually joined a local Toastmasters Club and restarted my education career by giving speeches on topics I was passionate about, including forest work, love, kindness.

As I completed that phase of healing, I hit another positive sign when I met my partner and best friend, Jenny. She was the first person in my life who I was completely honest with — and that remains to this day. I knew shortly after we connected that she would be in my life forever because I needed her friendship and support.

We were friends for several months before we had a chance and unexpected in-person meeting — and when the electricity went to another level, we decided to take the relationship from friends to dating.

I realized that with Jenny I *was truly in love for the first time*; all those past relationships were nothing compared to this one. Her love further helped my healing, expanding my heart and truly understanding the value and importance of self-love first, and then that deep love of a partner.

With Jenny's help, the next phase of my healing was reconnecting with my God… and it was through her church that my faith fully returned and grew… and still deepening today. I identify as a Christian, but I cringe sometimes stating that because so many hard-right Christians, so full of hate and not love, have really put a negative spin on people's perceptions of Christianity; so sad.

Interestingly, after several years traveling the country in our own version of "Van Life," we moved to a little forested hilltop, and are both actively working in this forest to bring it back to health.

The last step of my healing journey has been through the intentional use of psychedelics. I have had several healing (macro/full-dose) journeys, with both psilocybin and Ayahuasca, bringing my healing journey to a good place, especially in my spiritual healing journey and in my ego healing journey. When I intentionally consume psychedelics, I usually take a strong dose to help get right to what I need to see to heal.

I have also consumed LSD, but its work is more inspirational and empowering — but maybe that's still part of healing? LSD inspired my recent book, *Triumph Over Trauma*, and my foray forward with this healing project... so, in a sense, the medicine is helping with healing!

My healing is maintained through living these healing modalities — in maintenance form.

In other words, here is what I do to maintain my health:

- Eat farm-fresh or organic foods
- Spend time in nature often
- Consume several health supplements
- Pray or meditate daily
- Take multiple mindfulness/gratitude moments daily
- Occasionally microdose a psychedelic; would do a macrodose if something arose
- Take medicinal cannabis for pain, sleep
- Starting a focus on energy flows, chakras, tapping
- Ongoing integration of my healing

Final Words of Advice

Here's my suggestions for how you can start your healing journey:

- Believe that you are worthy — deserving — of healing.
- Start researching these healing modalities to find the ones that resonate with you.
- Find a coach, therapist, and community; you need people who have healed to help you on your healing journey.
- Try one or more of these healing modalities — maybe more than once.
- Plan to spend the rest of your life integrating the healing lessons, maintaining your healing, and learning more about yourself.

Editor's Notes About Ran's Healing Journey

- Comparison Syndrome is a real issue — whether we are comparing our strengths or our traumas. Instead, we must really focus inwardly, and concentrate on our healing.
- Wearing multiple masks — so-called personality masks allow us to hide our true selves from others — is definitely a sign that you need healing. Wearing masks is exhausting, but allows us to protect the true, inner self from more hurt.
- While other healing modalities get more attention, healing through communing and appreciating nature can be extremely powerful.
- Psychedelic substances, especially plants and fungi, have truly amazing effects on the brain, allowing for powerful healing when done with intention and followed up with integrating the experience.
- To truly find yourself again — and then maintain that healing — you need to keep using these modalities. Healing takes work and time, and the healing journey is never really over.

CHAPTER 21:
Healing Journey Story #2

Healing Requires Radical Responsibility

First Name: Daphne

Age: Generation X

Gender: Female

Why I started on my healing journey: To counterbalance my stressful and competitive day job.

Words that describe where I am on my healing journey: Constantly dancing toward death.

Most valuable thing you've learned on your healing journey: Radical responsibility for self.

Progress on your healing journey: Leader of my own life.

Hardest part of your healing journey: Resisting addiction and overcoming miseducation around "drugs."

Best advice to someone just starting their healing journey: Find circles of healing that welcome you, or start them yourself.

My Healing Story:

When I look back at my life, I can see I've always been on a healing journey. But I didn't always call the activities "healing." It's only recently that I started seeing them that way.

Since early childhood, I've felt a need for movement. In elementary school, it was gymnastics and Scottish dancing. In high school, it was tennis and cross country and horseback riding. I didn't like to compete; I just liked to play and move.

Movement was healing for me, though I didn't realize it, and children's activities aren't really set up like that. Parents and coaches entered me in the tennis tournament, the gymnastics meet, the highland dance competition. I never won ribbons or trophies, but that wasn't why I was there. I found safety, strength, and flexibility in my body.

When I graduated from journalism school and moved to Toronto to take a newspaper job, I went to my first yoga class. That began a whole era. As the big city journalist's lifestyle began to become clear to me — *toxic, sedentary, and stressful* — I committed further to a regular practice.

I needed yoga spaces, people, and mindsets to counterbalance the male-dominated workplaces and competitive mindset that permeated the field I had chosen. Yoga was my way of accessing my feelings, my feminine self, my inner teacher.

By going to yoga classes after work — instead of going drinking with my colleagues — I cultivated alternatives to the alcohol-oriented social opportunities that were everywhere around me. I found a woman-friendly community.

I also found social healing in Toronto's rave community. The people and social norms in the rave community of the late 1990s and early 2000s were more fem-friendly than those of nightclubs.

MDMA and the culture around it were incredibly important to me for a while. I danced, I made friends, I processed the sexism I was experiencing in the work world. I hadn't had the whole picture of what it meant to be a female adult before, and now I could see things from a new perspective.

I became more me and less what other people expected of me. I could see the good in myself and in the people around me. Music sounded better than ever before.

I felt freedom in my female body. I could be beautiful, and I could offer and celebrate my own beauty as a gift to a non-binary universe rather than as a high-priced trap for the male gaze. There were no dance competitions or performance expectations, it was free movement for its own sake.

Over time, I found that raves were a substance minefield and therefore, full of relationship drama. The vibe changed over time, and I moved away, but my community stuck with me. The circles of friends that now surround me have roots that stretch back to the rave scene, and the people I met there have been a huge part of my healing. My husband is one of them.

During that time in my career, I developed a relationship with a yoga ashram located in British Columbia, Yasodhara Ashram. It's located on a beautiful piece of land, on a lake, in the mountains. It's led by women, and worshipping the Divine Feminine is an organizing principle.

I appreciate the teachers and teachings at Yasodhara so much, and the land and nature are so healing for me. Over a 20-year period, Yasodhara has become my spiritual home. I can go there on my own and I know I will meet up with familiar people, and I'll also meet some new people.

The ashram has a great karma yoga program for young people and the community has a healthy influx of new folks, while also having a consistent community of elders and teachers. That makes it a very attractive place for me, and I hope to have a relationship with Yasodhara as I age.

Other healing methods:

Reflective writing, fiction writing, and expressive art therapy are other healing practices that have helped me over the years. In these realms I have found and created circles of women who wish to create intentional and intersectional circles of support.

My various circles of healing women may *look* like a networking group, a knitting meetup, or a book club, but *actually*, we worship the Divine Feminine in each other, share spells and pool resources in preparation for a revolution.

I became interested in psychedelics as another healing avenue for myself about two years ago. During the pandemic, like everyone, I had some trauma. Mine looked like medical trauma.

I guess it had been sort of building up. My husband had suffered a concussion in 2016 and the symptoms were disabling. He wasn't able to work, socialize, exercise, or do much of anything. He had no stamina and was very sensitive to sound and light and motion.

Doctors did not really do anything to help him. That was frustrating for him, and for me. He eventually found someone in the U.S. who was doing concussion treatment differently and started to feel better just as the pandemic began. It took us all a while to believe he was better.

Then, near the beginning of the pandemic, my son, who was 11, had some seizures. It took a while to recognize them and get a medical appointment with a pediatric neurologist. Then he was diagnosed with epilepsy with no known cause.

The whole experience of my son's diagnosis was overlaid with the pandemic. The doctor, who had terrible manners, gave us the news on the phone. When we did meet her for a few minutes, we all had masks on. We eventually moved to a different doctor, but the recommended treatment was the same — daily drugs.

It was extremely alienating to be given the diagnosis and then referred to a non-profit for resources. The non-profit wasn't very helpful. I tried reaching out to friends on Facebook, but those who responded weren't very helpful either, as there are so many different types of epilepsy and it seemed no one had similar experiences to us.

When I started researching epilepsy, I had a strong intuition that my son's condition had epigenetic causes that came through me and linked back to my mother.

I started researching everything about epilepsy, and I personally believe that my intuition is right, but the medical world doesn't really "treat" epigenetic causes of epilepsy. They just give pharmaceuticals. I find that to be an oversight.

I decided I needed to heal myself as a way of healing the epigenetic causes that might be affecting my son's health. I knew I had to be able to better manage the stress of not knowing when my son might have a seizure. I knew I needed to be able to care for myself so that when he has seizures, I can stay calm.

My interest in healing the brain and the nervous system made my ears perk up when friends first started talking about microdosing a few years ago. They were mostly men, though, and they were doing it to be more productive at work. That didn't interest me much, I have to admit.

Additional healing:

But I was thoroughly convinced that psychedelics might hold healing potential for me when I attended a spiritual cannabis retreat with guidance from psychotherapists and a plant elder in a natural setting.

I had used cannabis many times and, in my mind, it was a recreational experience. Sure, smoking a joint could be a fun and sensorially pleasing good time, but the cannabis retreat was a profoundly moving experience.

Being at a retreat center and in the care of a plant elder felt more like a yoga retreat than a rave, and I began to see how my yoga experiences and my use of mind-altering substances could come together in a responsible way.

Parts of me that were formerly separate were somehow unified on that retreat. I realized there was so much I didn't know about cannabis and psychedelics. I gained appreciation for the three-part psychedelic process — intention, ceremony, and integration.

For me, this process is even more important than whatever substance or dosage I might choose to ingest. The substance actually seems secondary to me. Psychedelics are a process, not a pill.

They're a whole story with a beginning, a middle, and an ending that reveals how the characters have changed. They're much more than a climax.

I am drawn to learn more about psilocybin next, and eventually other psychedelics in a more intentional, ceremonial way than I have used these substances in my party past.

Just as with cannabis, I suspect I've been miseducated about the potential of mushrooms, ayahuasca, and mescaline. I'm particularly interested in plants as medicine, and the chemical psychedelics like LSD and ketamine don't interest me as much. Psychedelics as a way of communicating with nature appeals to me greatly.

My intention with psychedelics is to face my fear of discomfort. My intention is to face my resistance to the realities of life, such as pain, loss, and death. My intention is to go deeper into my own wisdom than ever before.

I'm definitely interested in doing a large dose of psilocybin, but I'm also really curious about medium doses. This is an area of psychedelic practice that I feel is not really talked about, but it should be. Microdosing and macrodosing dominate the conversation.

I would like to get to know the medium dose so that I can combine psychedelics with yoga, expressive arts such as dancing, painting, and writing, and nature walks. I'm now getting training for psychedelic facilitation and integration coaching so that I can offer these experiences to others.

I'm also really interested to know more specifics about how psychedelics may or may not be used by people who have specific health conditions:

- Can someone with epilepsy use them?
- Can someone who has concussion symptoms benefit from them?
- What about epigenetics? How might psychedelics affect our genes through the generations?

- What about young people? How might teens use or not use these substances? What have traditional societies that use psilocybin been speaking about and doing with their children? This is a blind spot in Western approaches to psychedelics in my opinion.

The subject of children and psychedelics is extremely ethically loaded, but we need to talk about it so that everyone has access to healing and access to knowledge about whether it would be safe for them.

Still, I see psychedelics are but one color in a rainbow of healing possibilities. The first line of treatment is, I clean my house. Then I get some exercise. Then, I call a friend. I write some affirmations. I drink a glass of water. Then I get intimate with my husband. Then, *maybe* a psychedelic journey?! Or maybe not. Like I said, it's garnish, not a meal.

Healing Insight:

When I have experienced backslides or bumps on my healing journey, I have found that I can return to my body any time I need. It's always there for me, ready to reveal wisdom I already own.

My most trusted practices are yoga and reflective writing. I return to these practices because they cost nothing and can be done alone or with friends in natural settings.

The most valuable thing I've learned on my healing journey is that it's up to me. When I take responsibility for my everyday choices, healing is available to me.

This kind of radical responsibility is sometimes difficult to face. But it's also empowering. I don't need to pay a teacher or buy a product. I don't need to study scripture or follow specific practices. I have what I need.

The hardest part of my healing journey has been letting go of the people who don't come with me on the healing journey.

When friends are using substances in unhealthy ways, I get very involved in their struggles. It is sometimes difficult to maintain boundaries. But my belief that every person must take responsibility for their own healing requires me to invest fully in my own choices, and to accept the choices others make for themselves.

My advice to people who are on their healing journey is to commit to a process of intention, ceremony, and integration. Understand what those words mean to you, and start to live them every day. Find practices and people who are readily accessible to you.

Let go of the idea that products, pills, places, or plants can heal you. Only you can heal you, and only practices and people can help.

Community is essential for true growth and healing. Look for circles of people who are gathering to heal and who are actively supporting each other's journeys.

Final Words of Advice

If you don't currently have a safe circle of folks who welcome you and make you feel safe, keep looking. Keep reaching out. Create a circle of two or three people and be welcoming to newcomers. Show up for others as a way of showing up for yourself. Show people how you want to be treated by encouraging them and helping them.

Editor's Notes About Daphne's Healing Journey

- Community is an essential part of the healing journey. While a healing journey is an individual experience, the journey can be so much stronger, supported, and enhanced through the support and feedback from trusted friends.
- A hallmark of a healing journey is taking ownership — perhaps for the first time — of your life, your healing, your health.
- A key realization along the healing journey is that you already have all the tools you need to heal within you; you don't need a magic pill to heal, but you do need to commit to finding the healing modalities that work best for your healing — and then doing the work to truly heal.
- Physical movement — somatics — is a key healing modality for — and combining music with dance makes it an even more special tool for many.
- Even when consumed recreationally, psychedelic medicines can result in healing and growth, but it is best to be intentional, to do the medicine work in a safe setting, and follow up with the much-needed integration of the experiences.

CHAPTER 22:
Healing Journey Story #3

The True Path

First Name: Louisa

Age: Gen Z

Gender: Female

How/Why You Started on Healing Journey: I studied psychology for years. This was my dream and I started working full-time, but the job made me really unhappy and led to unhealthy decisions and self-medicating.

Words That Describe Where You are in Your Healing Journey: In the process of still integrating healing experiences. Still thinking of things I was allowed to see and I experienced. Thinking of them every day.

Most Valuable Thing You've Learned on Your Healing Journey: "Nothing is as you think it is." There are so many things inside us that we can't access in our daily life. So many things that need to stay subconscious in order to keep us functioning.

Progress on Your Healing Journey: Still figuring out what makes me happy. Expressing myself creatively everyday (on LinkedIn for example). Exploring the world. Meeting new inspiring people. Choosing each day how I want my life to be. Travelling the world, experiencing life.

Hardest Part of Your Healing Journey: Seeing some of the trauma of my past when I wasn't ready for it. It was also quite hard to quit my old job, because it gave me a lot of stability—and it had been my "dream" job. It was so hard to listen to myself. I was always told to do what others told me.

Best Advice to Someone Just Starting Their Healing Journey: Don't force yourself to heal. Healing will happen organically. It's a lifelong process.

My Healing Story:

My path to healing started with talk therapy when I was 17 to try and help the depression I suffered with since I was 14. The therapy helped explain why I had a lot of problems during my teen years, but never got to the root of the cause.

After my therapy, which went on for one and a half years, I decided to travel to Australia and New Zealand for a while.

After traveling, I still had depressive episodes.

At the time, I knew I wanted to study psychology and become a psychotherapist. I hadn't taken any drugs or psychedelics at this time. I started studying and knew I didn't have the energy or mental capacity to finish the work because I was depressed all of the time.

I decided to go back to therapy. My second round of therapy sessions went more in depth into my childhood and the trauma I experienced. I went to my second therapist for more than 5 years. It went so deep that at times, I felt like I couldn't handle it anymore. In psychology, we say I 'decompensated.' This is why I took antidepressants for 2 years.

Things from my childhood came up in therapy that made me feel really uncomfortable. In the beginning, it was so intense that I couldn't leave the house or talk to people. I got paranoid and felt so unsafe. But with the ongoing therapy and medication, I felt I could handle it (or push it down).

But because I had pushed down that childhood trauma, the symptoms of depression became worse and worse — while I was in therapy.

As an adult, I now I know I wasn't ready to deal with certain things when I was a child. I was too young to understand when the abuse happened.

I finished my therapy. The antidepressants did help me deal with my trauma, anxiety, and a lot of anger that came to the surface during the therapy. And in general, after therapy, I felt a lot better ... but I also I stopped taking the antidepressants.

The therapy and medications kept me functioning; otherwise I wouldn't have finished my studies.

At the end of my studies, I got into recreational drugs (including alcohol). I am not sure why, but maybe to deal with my therapy ending.

Once I graduated, I started working as a psychologist. During this time, I managed to party and do drugs only on the weekends — and thus, I was still good at my job. But deep down, I wasn't feeling happy.

I didn't really understand why I was unhappy in my career field. I studied psychology for years and was so looking forward to working in the field — but I just didn't like my job.

I always thought I did everything right, per society's rules: I went to therapy and did all the work that needed to be done, but it felt like my brain didn't show me what I needed to see.

Maybe I subconsciously sensed psychedelics offered me what I felt was the missing piece of the puzzle. I tried out ketamine, LSD, and magic mushrooms (psilocybin). But I never consumed the psychedelics alone; close friends were always there to support me.

Taking psychedelics for healing was not really planned. I was just exploring and experimenting with them. I did LSD several times (macrodosing). But I also have a history with alcohol and drugs and I have tried everything. I also did a lot of ketamine, but it did nothing to help me with my healing journey.

Before I started my healing journey unintentionally, I didn't really know I was unhappy — I thought, *I am healed*. I didn't think of changing my life. I was just having fun with psychedelics.

But I quickly discovered there were still things left, things the psychedelics allowed me to explore and heal. I didn't really think there was anything left to discover, but psychedelics proved me wrong.

Taking psychedelics felt like several intense therapy sessions combined — and I was *not* prepared for that because I was taking them recreationally, rather than with intent. And I mean intense — not in a positive way, but more in a cruel and necessary way.

I remembered things years back in my childhood that I had completely pushed away — heavy things — issues people shouldn't be going through alone. In my opinion, this is why we need psychedelics included in therapy and to not leave people alone with trauma they can't handle on their own.

I discovered I had pushed away sexual abuse from my childhood, burying it deeply inside; otherwise, I would have collapsed as a child or young teenager.

I saw during two LSD trips that my patients were my own mother. The whole time I was working with them, I was actually trying to help my mom (subconsciously). I wanted to help her and make her feel better, but I couldn't do it. (She is a chronic alcoholic — for years now.)

I reached a point in which I couldn't work in my job as a psychologist anymore; it was too much pressure, I encountered triggering situations, and I felt I couldn't help the people who were coming to me.

Because of my psychedelic experiences, I was allowed to see who I want to be, how I want to feel, and how being alive can feel. The feeling of being connected to my own energy is something I try to remember every day.

Here's what I have learned on my healing journey:

1. I learned that I was unhappy in my job as a psychologist — and I could change that. I worked in a very difficult field with adults suffering from chronic mental health conditions (where there is no hope left for being healed). This made me sad and depressed, because I felt I couldn't help. I saw these people suffer every day.
2. I learned you can change anything. If you're unhappy, you're in control of changing things. I finally quit my job and did a lot of other things (working on retreats, starting LinkedIn, writing and content creation, etc.). Life is about making choices for yourself, doing what's in your best interest. Just because you were on a certain path for a while, you don't need to stay on that path. Choose a life that makes YOU happy

3. Because of psychedelics, I learned that I need to help myself, take care of myself. I cannot help everyone. Furthermore, If I feel unhappy I am allowed to change it.

Healthy, healing habits:

I now include meditation and yin yoga in my daily life because it's a way of being connected to my true self and my true path in life. The progress of healing comes from allowing ourselves to have a look inside and listen to ourselves. We can only heal if we never let this connection disappear.

The psychedelics showed me I am allowed to do what I want. The hardest part was not only to quit my job but also to know *why* I needed to quit. I now know the reason why I became a psychologist. But the reason didn't make me happy. I was trying to heal my mom. Each client was a part of my mom I wanted to heal. I tried my best. I couldn't help everyone. I realized some people don't want help (like my mom), and I needed to accept it.

The hardest part of psychedelics is being confronted with things we usually don't know — trauma that comes up and we have to deal with it. This is difficult.

I am in still the process of integrating what I experienced on LSD. I learned a lot through psychedelics. They offered me a different view of myself. They are **not** a magic pill; they do not result in some magical transition where everything is now great.

We always need to put in the work afterward. The more intense the trip, the harder the integration will be.

Every day, I am thinking of things I was allowed to see and experience. This is why I haven't done LSD since my last intense trip in November. I am still processing and integrating… talking and sharing with close friends and family members.

Key words of advice:

If you don't feel ready for psychedelics, don't take them. You need to be willing to be confronted with the truth → there is no way back! Some people don't want that confrontation. And some people don't want to go to therapy. Psychedelics are NOT fun. They have a lot of potential, but they can be scary as well.

Integration and Future Plans:

I am choosing actions mindfully and aligned with the insights I gained (via yin yoga, meditation, long walks, etc.). And honestly, I am still overwhelmed. I am not planning on doing anything new in the future — except perhaps microdosing for further integration. But I am still integrating and expressing my creativity and doing some more traveling — to Bali and then Vietnam.

Final Advice:

Life is about making the choices you want. Just because you are on a certain path for a while, you don't need to stay on that path. Choose a life that makes YOU happy.

Because of psychedelics, I discovered I cannot help everyone. I need to help myself, take care of myself. If I feel unhappy, I am allowed to change it.

Don't force yourself to heal. Healing will happen organically. It's a journey, a lifelong process. Healing will happen when the timing is right — when you're strong enough to see what you need to see to truly heal.

Editor's Notes About Louisa's Healing Journey

- All healing journeys have ebbs and flows, periods of great healing and periods of struggle. Again, the key is simply being aware that the healing journey will not always be a positive one, and you will face hurdles — but you have the tools to overcome all obstacles and find that place of truth, love, and joy.
- Psychedelic medicines may or may not play a role in your healing journey, but if you are considering using them as one of your healing modalities, it's best to take them in a safe setting — with a supportive community and/or with a willing therapist or coach. Note that recreational use of psychedelics can quickly become an unexpectedly intense experience.
- You are in control of your life, and one of the greatest benefits from true healing of past trauma is understanding yourself, perhaps for the first time. Too often, we let others define us, but when we heal, we live our true/authentic lives.
- So many of us have been adversely affected by childhood trauma — whether we actually remember it or have buried it deeply inside. The key to healing is understanding that trauma (as an adult), forgiving yourself (and the abuser), and integrating all aspects of the healing journey — for as long as it takes.

CHAPTER 23:
Healing Journey Story #4

Be Wholly Human

First Name: TJ

Age: Millennial

Gender: Male

How/Why You Started on Healing Journey: I was chasing external accomplishments thinking they would bring lasting happiness and fulfillment. After 12 years of general success in the military and corporate world, I understood that it was a path to emptiness. As I was working full-time and enrolled in a full time MBA program, I watched the fall of Afghanistan all over the news. It was the darkest place of my life as I watched something that was once my life's purpose crumble in front of my eyes. I was depressed and had frequent suicidal thoughts. It was then I knew I needed to make changes. I didn't know what I was looking for, but I started moving toward it.

Words That Describe Where You are in Your Healing Journey: I am elevating and sharing the journey.

Most Valuable Thing You've Learned on Your Healing Journey: Our inner world drastically impacts how we view the outer world, and that's a choice. Life is a game of overcoming fear to break mental patterns that keep us stuck in cycles that are not serving us. By exploring and accepting our own shadow, that which we don't want to show the world, we become free.

Progress on Your Healing Journey: It's been beautiful. I feel as though I am just getting started.

Hardest Part of Your Healing Journey: The fear and negative emotions that come with breaking upper limits and holding the space.

Best Advice to Someone Just Starting Their Healing Journey: Everything you think and feel is ok. Do not be afraid of those negative emotions. They will come in waves you can handle. The air is always cleaner after those storms. See the beauty in it, and those roots will grow deep. It's so worth it.

My Healing Story:

I was in the Marine Corps for eight years as an infantry officer. I did three deployments, one to Afghanistan, one on a naval vessel, and then one to Japan and Korea. After my service in the Marines, I transitioned to the corporate world, where I worked in medical device sales for four years.

Both were great experiences, tons of lessons learned. And after four years working in medical device sales, I transitioned and moved on to this, which is stepping into coaching. And so much of this change is integrated with my healing journey. So perhaps before I talk about the healing journey, I'll talk a little bit more about the road that led me to the point where I was like, "Oh my goodness, where am I right now?"

I was born and raised on Long Island, New York. Very much a blue-collar, middle-class town. I played sports, had a bunch of really good friends, many of whom I'm still friends with. September 11th, 2001, was a day that affected so many of us — and it affected me deeply. My best friend's dad, who was also our baseball coach and just an all-around great guy, was a firefighter with Ladder 118 and he passed away on 9/11. There's actually a very moving photo of a firetruck going across the Brooklyn Bridge toward the burning towers, and that was their rig. That was the last photo snapped of him and his crew.

I remember coming home from school that day, and I just stood in front of the TV for... for what seemed to be hours, just staring at the images of the burning towers, the replay of the planes crashing into the building, and confusion, anger, so many emotions.

I knew then that I was going to join the military. So fast forward nine years, I graduated high school, but I was 17, so I couldn't enlist in the Marines without my mom's permission. She did not give me permission. So I went to college and did ROTC (Reserve Officers' Training Corps) and played lacrosse. And the day I graduated was the day I was commissioned as a second lieutenant in the Marine Corps.

It was incredible experience to be able to lead and serve with great people; it is an honor that I will always cherish. About a year after getting to my first unit, we deployed to Afghanistan. The area I was in wasn't a very kinetic area; there wasn't a lot of fighting.

At the time, I thought I wanted the fighting.

I thought that's what I needed to prove myself: to go and fight every day and to take it back to the enemy, the people who perpetrated 9/11 or the people who harbored the people who perpetrated 9/11. I have this moment that I now reflect on when I was in Afghanistan; it was December 24th, and there was a marine in a sister company who was killed on December 23rd. And he was a great man. I didn't know him, but everything I've heard about Sergeant Danny Basilian is that he's just one of those people that people gravitated toward... a true leader. And so we were told that we couldn't patrol on December 25th, meaning we couldn't leave the wire on December 25th because it would be too difficult for family members to receive news that their son or daughter was killed on Christmas.

And that was the first time it hit me: we're at war here. So... human life is human life. What does it matter if we die on December 25th or January 1st? But I wasn't able to look deeply into that. It was just this underlying feeling of, wow, what's going on?

I got back from that deployment and I felt just as unfulfilled as before I left, because I had this idea that if I went to combat, one of two things would happen. One, I would prove myself in this ultimate, ultimate crucible of a life test, and I would have fulfillment and pride and admiration for the rest of my life, right? I had proved myself to myself. Or, two, I would die.

And in a way, while I was never in a life or death situation, I liked the idea of it. I welcomed it because my ego was saying, "die a hero, be remembered."

What better way to go out, you know? And then I wouldn't have to deal with this underlying anger and these emotions that I buried, just as so many kids do or young people do. Alcohol, you know, whatever substance it is. I was self-medicating for much of my life, and alcohol was a big part of that.

I got back home from that deployment and felt empty. And I was thinking, okay, well let's try to get back to a deployment that may lead to combat. So I volunteered for another deployment and didn't go to combat. A couple more years, one more deployment, didn't go to combat, but I started to get this sense that maybe what I was looking for, I wasn't going to find in the Marines. I didn't know what that was, but I just started to get this idea that maybe it's not there.

So I transitioned out of the Marine Corps, and again, very grateful for the experiences and the lessons learned. I mean, I developed a love for nature, which I'll talk more about, and the people that I served with — truly selfless people who put others above themselves at some level. And I think that needs to be honored and cherished.

I landed a job with a great company working in medical device sales. I started making more money and I thought, okay, I served for eight years.... Now it's time to live the American dream. And I saw the next 25, 30 years in front of me, never having to worry about money, right? So if I don't have to worry about that and I could live this life of kind of upscale life, I felt, all right, this is it.

I was still striving for the external accomplishments, so I enrolled in an MBA program a year later. I'm working full-time and in a full-time MBA program. The more I accomplished, the more I realized those accomplishments weren't going to bring me what I was looking for. But I didn't know what I was looking for, so I just kept going.

So... I am working full-time, in a full-time MBA program, and then the images of the Afghan withdrawal are all over the news. And it just crushed me. It crushed me because what was once my life's purpose, what I thought was going to bring me that meaning, was now crumbling in front of my eyes. And I was angry, I was sad, I was confused... and I was still showing up to work every day with a smile on my face.

But that was the darkest time of my life.

I had suicidal thoughts. There was a night when I was drunk and I had my loaded AR-15 next to me and pointed at me, safety off. I don't know if I would've done it, but it just gave me this sense of control... I could end this if I want to.

When I woke up the next day and I thought, "Oh shit, I'm that guy. I'm there. There's no more pretending. You are at that point."

So over the next couple of months, my marriage wasn't in a good place and so much of that is me not being able to work through my own challenges. So my ex-wife and I split. Now I'm alone with myself — for the first time in eight years in the house that we shared.

I decided I can go one of two ways. I can go back to the TJ in his early twenties, partying, except now with a little more money in my pocket, so I could go to Vegas, Miami, all that. And I did a little of that during the last year too. Or I can go this other path, which is something different.

I didn't know what I was looking for, but it was something different. I started running and started with five miles, then another five miles, then 10 miles. One day I decided that I'm going to run 30 miles. And so I did — and it was ugly and it was slow and it was painful. But I finished that 30 mile run/walk and I just had this underlying feeling of joy for the first time in a long time... I didn't need anyone else or anything else.

I just needed to believe in something that I could do and then do it. Running became a foundation of healing for me.

I also found a therapist who I connected with. Therapy is so important, yet I hadn't found a therapist with whom I truly connected until this time. Therapy, too, was another foundation for healing. Having someone to share these experiences with, who understood what I was going through and basically be there to reflect back, "Hey, you're not crazy. It's okay to have these thoughts."

I'm grateful for my therapist and we are still close friends. Shout out if she reads this one day.

Then I had this urge: I had to get away from where I was — at the house that my ex-wife and I shared — so I went out and I did a four-day solo camping trip in Asheville, North Carolina.

When I was in the Marines, I read this book, *The Power of Now*, by Eckhart Tolle, but I wasn't in a place where I could read it with an open heart. When I did read it, I had this glimpse of seeing things from a different perspective. On this camping trip, as I sat on the grass one day after a nice long run for about four or five hours, I decided if people can meditate, I was going to figure this out. Why can't I do this?

It was this intense surrender, so to speak, because it's really uncomfortable to be in your own thoughts — very uncomfortable. Finally, after many hours, I started to get some space between my thoughts, observe them, and feel the energy in my body and then feel that energy merge with the energy of nature around me.

I opened my eyes; I had tears coming down and I looked out at the mountains and the trees and I just saw it in a way deeper than I'd ever seen it before. And it was this understanding that everything is already perfect. I was raised Catholic and I was baptized as an adult. I tried to understand the teachings of Jesus

— and in that moment, it made more sense than ever before. That was a pivotal point because I realized there's more depth to me. I'm starting to understand this.

Again, I went back to "normal" life. I was working, I got into another relationship that was kind of up and down at the time. Old patterns, and again, that's on me. But I still wasn't aware of how to get out of those old patterns... how to break them.

I ran my first ultramarathon a couple of months later, and the night before, I had a dream about my dad that was very powerful but I didn't really act on it.

Then last December, I was again at this point where I felt it's okay, I know that there's more to this, but I'm still in the same patterns and routines at work, in relationships, and with myself. I knew I needed to get away again.

I was actually considering going down to Peru to do an Ayahuasca retreat. It felt rushed though, and I was a bit intimidated to get on a plane and go down there — because I understand the immense power and beauty of plant medicine and psychedelics. I'd never done psychedelics up to that point. It didn't feel right; it felt rushed.

Instead I went to the desert by myself... to Big Bend National Park (in Texas). I had this Airbnb for five days and drove out to the park. I'm sitting in silence, no cell phone service. I brought enough coffee for one cup of coffee per day and all the food and water I needed... and my running shoes. I was so uncomfortable and had these feelings that no one cares if you're here, so just leave. *No one cares.* But I made a deal with myself to run 20 miles per day for four days.

I started to get very much in tune with the rhythm of nature. It was wonderful. I would go to sleep without looking at my phone. I didn't even know what time it was. I'd wake up when it was still dark, but I was fully rested and I would go outside and sit and feel the night energy around me.

The moment the first ray of sunlight came over the mountains, the energy would shift to the day energy and the birds would start chirping. And it was bright and light and it's just, gosh, nature is perfect. It's all right here. It's wonderful.

On the third night, I was very much in tune and I was lying underneath the stars, the most beautiful night sky that I've ever seen... looking up at the Milky Way, focusing on my breath.

Suddenly, as I was looking at the stars, I noticed the darkness between the stars that popped out toward me. My heart started beating a little bit faster, as I pondered what is that? And I just kept breathing, kept breathing. I decided to surrender to it, let it happen. And that darkness came and it merged with my energy. It came all the way to me and it just felt like warmth and truth. And it was comfort. It just felt like comfort. It just made sense.

The next day when I woke up, I was even more in tune with the rhythm of nature. I was able to touch plants and feel my energy flow to it. Then it was late afternoon and I felt as though I was just sending my love out to this entire valley of plants and having a great time, like a child, with childlike joy.

I couldn't remember a time feeling that much pure joy since I was a kid.

When I looked at this mountain — or what appeared to be a dormant volcano in the distance — I used my energy and looked at it and I commanded it to erupt. And it didn't erupt. So I realized you probably can't bring things into this world that are bad for other people. I went back to singing and dancing to Incubus. But then, 45 minutes later, I was cooking dinner and it was a clear sky and I saw some smoke billowing from this distant mountain; I don't think it's actually a dormant volcano.

Oh my goodness. I was in denial and complete belief — simultaneously. *I just laughed.* And it was so beautiful. I'm not implying that I made that volcano smoke. Perhaps it would've happened anyway. But just being in tune with nature; for those that knock, the door will be opened and a deeper understanding is available. I don't know exactly what it means, but it made sense and it was beautiful.

So I left the desert after five wonderful days of camping, and I had to come back to New York for a wedding a couple weeks after that. During that trip, the opportunity to experience DMT came up — and I knew it was right.

The experience was beautiful. I took one inhale and I looked at my childhood friend who was my guide for that experience, and his face turned immediately into patterns. And I remember saying, "thank you, thank you. You're that guide, aren't you?" I recognized his energy and then I looked up at the trees and the trees turned to patterns... and I surrendered. I said. "show me."

My spirit left my body. Moving quickly, as though it was pulled by a magnet on the other side of the universe. It moved infinitely far, infinitely fast. But I felt it go. Then I was suspended and this infinite canvas of everything and nothing... beautiful patterns that I can't explain.

Two days later, I went for a run, and during that run, I became overwhelmed with the sense of joy and peace... as though all of the work that I'd been doing up to that point was confirmed during that DMT experience. It's hard to explain, but none of it was a surprise...

I've already known this; it's all right here. And now it's known, but it's buried deep within.

That psychedelic experience accelerated my healing journey just a little bit. But I think it's so important to emphasize this to people that it's not an answer, or the answer, or the only way. It is just a way. And when you're ready for it, I think it becomes available if you're called to it rather than going and seeking it in a forced manner.

Two days later, I wrote in my journal about how I was in the canvas of existence and everything and nothing. *And it was perfect.* And how the material world got built only makes sense that a higher power built it. And it was built with love — because look around, it's so beautiful here and there's beauty in everything.

I felt like a medium in which to allow love to pass through the canvas into the material and the material to the canvas. That's it. Love is just truth. It's truth in that good and bad does exist and it's okay; good and bad exists within all of us, and it's okay. I also wrote that I don't believe we have free will when we're locked into our thoughts — although we think we do. Once we become the observer of our thoughts, however, that's when we can start to change these patterns that are not serving us.

From that point on, I was so in tune with my energy and while I was working at a great company with great people, I just knew that I could not keep working there day after day, being in front of Zoom calls, sitting in on sales meetings and stuff. It wasn't where I needed to be; it wasn't fulfilling me or allowing me to give my best self to the world.

Thus, about three weeks after the DMT experience, I told my boss that I was going to leave and quit. And I didn't have a master plan. I just had something I had to share. I told my boss and my boss's boss — and they've been very supportive, encouraging.

I knew I was moving on, but I didn't know what I was moving into. I just had to start sharing these experiences, this healing journey, growth, and a deeper level of understanding.

Since then, I've had a few more profound experiences, one that I think is very important to note, and that's working through a panic attack with breathwork.

I have always had these feelings of underlying anxiety, fight or flight, but I was self-medicating with alcohol, porn, processed foods — anything to not feel it. TV distracted me.

Now I'm at this point in my healing journey where I'm beginning to share things publicly and be vulnerable. I'm not self-medicating to the extent that I was... so one night I felt this dark energy coming into me and around me, and I was alone in my apartment in Dallas. It was these deep thoughts: *wow, we are so powerful because if we can observe our thoughts, we could change our thoughts. And if we could change our thoughts, we could change our own world.*

And if we could change our own world, how good do we actually want to make it? How good can we make our world for ourselves — because it's really comfortable to stay in old patterns, even if they aren't serving us?

So it was those deep thoughts and then doubt... *can you really hold this space and share these feelings? Are you who you really think you are?* Then this darkness came into my chest and I'd never felt anything that deep before. I was lying down and was able to calm down, keep breathing. I went through my nightly routine. I got up and my knees were shaking, my hands were shaking. I walked into my bathroom. I couldn't even look in the mirror, but I brushed my teeth and grabbed my blanket. I then laid back down, turned on Solfeggio Frequencies, and envisioned myself wrapped in love.

Even though I was going through an internal storm, externally I felt safe... and then I started feeling that inner storm start to dissipate. I started to feel a little bit lighter, and then I did some breathwork. I turned on a free Wim Hof breathwork session on YouTube. As I went through it, those dark feelings really started to release. And then it was all light; it was so light. I was completely out of my thoughts and into my body. And my body was on fire in a beautiful way. I envisioned it a brighter white. Just so bright. And I slept like a baby.

The next morning I woke up and thought, "oh my gosh — these negative feelings are going to come, but it's okay because they come in waves that we can handle and we just have to let them do their work and teach us how powerful and how strong we really are."

We have to build our foundation with whatever tools we need, such as diet, breathwork, cold plunging, psychedelics, exercise. And when the storms come, yeah, they may shake us a little bit, but they're here to show us how strong the foundation is. Once I realized how strong that foundation is for overcoming fears, I realized we could keep going and holding that space.

It's just belief in overcoming your own doubt or own limiting beliefs and it's a choice and we are all that powerful.

In terms of integrating my healing journey... as I was becoming more public with it, I was so disciplined. I felt I had to wake up and get in the cold shower and then journal for 30 minutes and then go for a run. And then, and then, you know what I'm saying? It was so regimented and set in routine.

As I've been talking to other people and learning and growing and building more trust with myself, I am getting better at trusting in my higher self that I have these tools and I use them when I know that I need them. I can decide, no, maybe this morning I'm not going to do anything; I'm going to go eat breakfast and then an hour later I'm going to get in the cold ocean or then I'll sit down and journal.

So, today, that's basically how I integrate; it is just being open to new ideas and new tools for the toolbox and leveraging the ones that I know work for me when I know that I need them. And the profound ones for me are nature, cold plunging, breathwork, running, and diet.

Healing Realization:

Our spirit doesn't age; our spirit is who we are as kids, who we are as adults. It's our spirit; it's eternal. I love my mom, love my dad. But my first memory in life is hiding in a closet while my parents were arguing with each other. No hard feelings; it's okay. We all have our own trauma patterns. So it's important to go back and heal from that deep inner child work where I put myself back in these scenes that are hard to think about — because when I was living in these scenes, I couldn't allow my full emotions to be expressed and released because it's about survival; we have to survive in that.

In the healing journey, I have been able to go back to those moments as me, TJ now at 33, and walk in and visualize myself, helping my younger self out of that closet and giving myself a hug... with the message, you are worthy, *you are loved.*

It's about giving myself what I didn't get at the time. And again, it's not about, oh, my mom is a great human being. My dad was a great human being. We're all humans here doing the best that we can, but that inner child work is so essential to healing.

Key Insight:

And that is why Jesus says, unless you become childlike, you will not see the kingdom of heaven or enter the kingdom of heaven (Matthew 18:2-4). That inner child, that childlike curiosity about the world, asking why, questioning our own beliefs, why we think the way we do — it's so important and it's such a beautiful thing.

Some Final Thoughts

I now understand that trauma is deeply rooted in our subconscious. It can be from generational trauma, childhood trauma, or events in adulthood. Healing means we accept our trauma and our past and choose to love ourselves anyway. Only then can we truly love the world around us.

My healing journey certainly hasn't been smooth. In and out of another relationship that wasn't healthy. Minor setbacks here and there. By and large it has been continuous though.

Editor's Notes About TJ's Healing Journey

- Know that doubt and self-limiting/negative thoughts can work their way through as you progress through your healing journey. The key is knowing it might happen and challenging those thoughts to get to the root of the issue.
- For most people, true healing — and the maintenance of that healing journey — will come through the use of multiple modalities. Keep experimenting to find the modalities that work best for you.
- Sound can play a major role in healing. Solfeggio Frequencies are used to open chakras and bring about various mental and physical health benefits, depending on the frequency used, with frequencies ranging from 174 Hz to 963 Hz. (Learn more here: https://lonerwolf.com/solfeggio-frequencies/)
- Feelings of being unfulfilled in your professional and/or personal lives is a clear sign that you need to start a healing journey to find the answers... and to find your true, authentic self, and the path you are meant to follow.

CHAPTER 24:
Healing Journey Story #5

From Pain to Purpose

First Name: Angela

Age: Millennial

Gender: Female

How/Why You Started on Healing Journey: To understand why I had been so sickly since I was a child; to get to the root cause of all my health issues.

Words That Describe Where You are in Your Healing Journey: I believe that healing is a constant ebb and flow. I have learned to accept that healing is a journey and not a destination as we are always growing, learning and evolving throughout our lives. I believe the further along we get the more we can help others, which is where I currently am.

Most Valuable Thing You've Learned on Your Healing Journey: The most valuable thing I've learned on my healing journey was also one of the hardest. In order to heal, I had to create the foundation of *believing* that I could heal — which was actually really challenging for me. I was so sick that every day I woke up feeling and wondering if today was going to be the day I was going to die... and I begged God to take me away from the pain and suffering.

Progress on Your Healing Journey: I am truly grateful for the amount of progress I have made over these last couple of years. I went from being on my deathbed to learning how to thrive again. I have accepted that there will always be setbacks but these setbacks have helped me propel forward. I have learned, unlearned, and continue to surrender what no longer serves me while keeping my heart open and trusting the process. The more compassion, love, space and patience I have given myself, the more miracles I have seen within me and that has restored my faith that we all have the ability to heal ourselves if we just get out of our own way.

Hardest Part of Your Healing Journey: The hardest part of my healing journey was giving myself the space and patience to do so. When I was at my sickest it seemed as if no matter what I did I kept getting sicker. I was losing my ability to eat almost all foods, socialize, exercise, and I was barely functional. I kept seeking different practitioners, trying different methods and nothing seemed to be working and at the same time I knew my nervous system was so wound up that I wasn't going to get well until I learned to surrender.

Best Advice to Someone Just Starting Their Healing Journey: The best advice I can give someone who is just starting out their journey is to understand that healing isn't linear. It's a multi-layered process and in order to fully heal, one must address their healing holistically and address the body, mind, and soul as a ***whole***. Also, it's very important to be your own advocate. Don't settle for a mediocre diagnosis — as most diagnoses are often symptoms of a deeper root cause.

My Healing Story:

I grew up in a small town in northeastern Pennsylvania, and as far as I can remember in my 38 years of being alive, I was always sick with some sort of mysterious illness but most of the time, there was no explanation and no diagnosis. Growing up in the country, I spent most of my childhood outdoors playing in the woods, climbing trees, and going camping. I was a cheerleader, dancer, and tennis player, and loved working out and being active. I also had a healthy social life, blessed with a lot of friends to hang out with.

However, despite always being happy, healthy, and full of life, I can also remember that I was always sick. I learned at a young age how to push through illness and be a highly functional, chronically ill person. I had chronic allergies; rashes, food reactions, food impactions, strep throat, fatigue, brain fog and hormone and neurological issues just to name a few. I lived at my doctors' offices and after every visit they just threw another prescription at my parents and sent us on our way.

There also was a lot of emotional dysfunction in my family. I had an abusive alcoholic father who struggled with his own demons, and when I was nine years old, he unexpectedly passed away while my mom and I were on vacation visiting family in California. Losing my father at such a young age completely shocked me and had a damaging effect on my nervous system.

When I look back on my childhood and knowing what I know now about trauma and its connection to illness, I believe that living in constant fear and emotional distress had suppressed my immune system and was actually the root cause to being chronically ill.

In 2003, I graduated high school and moved to Los Angeles for college. I was subconsciously hoping that removing myself from the trauma that surrounded me in Pennsylvania would help me get well. While my mystery health issues didn't completely go away like I had hoped, they were much more easily managed up until December 2011, during a very stressful time at work. I was in and out of the ER with neurological stroke-like symptoms and no tests could confirm any diagnosis. Once again, I was sent home to sit with my symptoms and a referral to see a psychiatrist to get evaluated for mental illness.

Over that whole year I felt sicker each day. I could barely function at work. I lost weight and had numbness and tingling down my arms, legs, and all over my head and face. I tried exercising, but it would exacerbate my symptoms. I went to cardiologists, neurologists, gastroenterologists, and finally, a therapist to help me manage the anxiety and panic attacks.

After multiple sessions with my therapist, I learned how much trauma I had stored in my body from childhood — and while my therapist was convinced all of these health issues were stress-induced, I continued to search for answers.

In December 2012, I finally received my first diagnosis of an autoimmune disease in my esophagus called *eosinophilic esophagitis*, caused by food allergies. Then in January 2013, I started working with an allergist. After getting several allergy panels, I learned I was allergic to everything I was eating, and for a brief moment felt some sort of relief. I then started steroid medications, proton-pump inhibitors, antihistamines — and I had to immediately change my diet.

But still something didn't feel right. I kept searching for answers.

A month later I noticed there were red stains on my bra, but assumed after I had a full year of blood tests and workups that if it was anything major, the doctors would have found it.

Unfortunately, it was wishful thinking that the bleeding would eventually stop.

Instead, things got worse, and in May 2013, I was unexpectedly diagnosed with breast cancer. It was such a traumatizing diagnosis, but in the same breath I felt relieved I discovered what was causing my body to go haywire the whole year prior... and also proud of myself for advocating for my health — even when doctors were telling me there was nothing wrong.

While I thought that my cancer was the root of what was causing all of my mysterious illness symptoms, I soon learned it was only the beginning. What I didn't know at that time was that my breast cancer journey would be the start of my greatest healing journey — and set the tone for the rest of my life.

After the cancer was removed, my health continued to spiral downward. During that time, I felt so defeated by my body and so misled by my doctors. In every appointment, they just wanted to blame everything on post-cancer syndrome — and again sent me off with a different prescription. Meanwhile my health anxiety was at an all-time high.

One day, in a newsletter from my cancer center, I saw that there was a monthly Reiki circle for cancer survivors and their loved ones. Reiki is a Japanese style of energy healing that promotes relaxation and stress reduction so the body can come back into balance naturally. I was so desperate for relief and I felt in my heart I needed to see what it was about.

Through Divine intervention that day, I was introduced to two Reiki practitioners who ultimately saved and changed my life. One of the practitioners took me under her wing and I worked with her privately every week for 9 months — and after DECADES upon DECADES of being on a journey of sickness, I finally understood the effects of my childhood trauma, all while learning how to connect with my soul and unlock my own spiritual gifts.

I went from being on a sickness journey to a journey of healing and wellness.

After each session, I experienced such profound unexplained miracles in my body… and little by little, all of my mysterious "post cancer" symptoms were magically disappearing. My labs and tests were finally coming back normal, my food allergies were reversing, and my eosinophilic esophagitis also went into remission.

This was such a profound life-changing experience for me that I became passionate about wanting to help others who were also struggling — which led me to leaving my 10 year career in fashion to turn my pain into purpose and become a Reiki practitioner.

Through this journey, I became passionate about diet and nutrition, crystals, meditation, visualization, and developing my childhood gifts as a clairvoyant medium. After completing my Reiki Level Two certification in May, 2015, I took a leap of faith and started my own Intuitive Reiki and Holistic Wellness Practice, where I created a tailored mind body and soul program for my clients to come back into balance so that they too could heal themselves naturally.

For several years my health remained stable, but during that time I noticed I started to get pain and tingling in my left arm that eventually got diagnosed as thoracic outlet syndrome — caused by my top cervical rib compressing my brachial plexus nerve and subclavian artery. This ultimately led to me needing to undergo a major surgery to remove my left cervical rib in April 2019.

One week before the surgery, four years after starting my Reiki practice, I finally received my Master Attunement and teacher certification. I remember feeling so happy that everything was being completed and I was looking forward to starting my new chapter as a Reiki Master Teacher.

Unfortunately, the surgery did not go well, and I suffered from multiple complications, one of them being a collapsed lung that put me into the critical care unit for almost two weeks. When I got home from the hospital, my nervous system started to decline and I ultimately became bed-bound because I could no longer stand or walk without fainting.

My doctors assured me it would get better as I healed, but month after month I kept getting worse and after 6 months of fainting spells and failed autonomic nervous system tests, I lost my driver's license, my ability to drive, my ability to work, and worst of all, all of my food allergies were coming back with a vengeance and I was having anaphylactic reactions after everything I was eating.

My nervous system was so activated and scared. All of the tools I had learned and successfully used in my own healing practice were no longer working. Once again, I felt like I was knocking on death's door with no doctor in sight to help me — and I was left to advocate for myself. Intuitively, I felt this journey was going to lead me back to my roots, and in January 2021, I was intuitively guided to leave Los Angeles and head back to Pennsylvania to get answers.

After almost 2 years of being diagnosed with every neurological disease with no root cause, and 32 years of mysterious symptoms, in one month of being "home," I finally got to the **ROOT** cause of every single diagnosis and symptom — including the breast cancer.

Finally, after 32 years of being chronically unwell, in February 2021, I received a diagnosis of late-stage neurological Lyme disease, coinfections bartonella and Babesia, and also mold toxicity. By this point I was so sick I once again thought I was going to die. My Lyme doctor said I was too sick to do treatments and left it to me to figure out how to get healthy without medication.

This process cracked me open to a new level of healing, learning, and unlearning. I had to go against everything I thought was possible to heal — like shifting from eating fruits and vegetables to eating a strict carnivore diet... because my body couldn't tolerate digesting plants or starch anymore. Since I could not take supplements or medications because I was so hyper sensitive, I put my head down and prayed for guidance.

I truly believe that nutrition sets the foundation of our healing, and since I became reactive to so many plants, I switched to the low histamine Carnivore Diet of only non-aged ruminate meat such as beef, lamb, goat, veal and venison, organs, fat, and salt. For more than 2 years, it has been the biggest game changer for my health — and has reversed so many of my neurological symptoms.

I found alternative medicine practitioners and did holistic therapies such as kinesiology, acupuncture, Reiki, pulsed electromagnetic field therapy (PEMF), hypnotherapy, and bio-resonance therapy. I also found a Lyme-literate naturopath who taught me about detoxing naturally using a dry brush and Epsom salt baths. I also used her infrared sauna several times a week.

I later found a biological dentist and addressed oral cavitations and found out one of my root canals was harboring black mold, which was another root cause of why I got so ill.

I bio-hacked with sunrises, sunsets, and grounding.

Most importantly, I worked on the trauma I experienced as a child and began healing the inner child wounds from the abuse and abandonment in her childhood home decades ago — and who was now back after all these years. Facing this trauma as an adult was difficult, and during this process my escape (aka, childhood friends) were all busy with their adult lives so I was forced to really sit and be present with myself and my feelings.

In the beginning, it was agony and I became very disassociated. The pain of it all made me become suicidal at times, and it took me into a vortex of the dark night of the soul.

During this transformative, dark, time, it taught me how to become my own best friend...it forced me to have difficult conversations with my mother, deep meditations reconnecting with my deceased father, and I began a practice of forgiving both of them — while forgiving myself for the years I allowed myself to carry it.

I learned, and continue to learn, the importance of practicing self-compassion, self-love, and self-care... and ultimately learned to not attach myself to my diagnosis and mindfully change the relationship I have with my symptoms.

After 6 months of hard work, patience, and dedication, my life started to shift in miraculous ways, and I went from being chronically bed-bound to being able to walk again to being able to drive again. As my healing journey continued, I got my body strong enough to start homeopathic treatments — and from April 2022 until March 2023, I treated the Lyme, Babesia, and Bartonella... and I began hiking again.

My journey is still in progress as I am learning that this disease can't be cured, but can be put into remission. I now additionally do biweekly colonics, monthly vitamin infusions, Reiki, yoga 3-5 days a week, and maintain a carnivore diet. I also walk every day, meditate daily, cook, listen to podcasts, hike once a week, and spend as much time in nature as I can — as a way to maintain my balance as I prepare to take on the next round of treatments.

During this time, I have also maintained my Remote Intuitive Reiki and Holistic Wellness Practice and as I expanded in my healing, I have helped others expand in theirs. I also now work mainly with a lot of people who are also going through Lyme, mold, and other autoimmune and chronic diseases.

Final Thoughts:

I'm still healing and learning as these infections unfold, I'm still making peace with the trauma of my childhood and forgiving the parts of my soul for the things it didn't know and honoring my body in the process. Healing is a true art so whether I'm taking time for myself to heal or I'm helping someone else as a practitioner, I am grateful to be at both ends of the spectrum now.

Thinking of Loss: One of the other things I struggled with — and continue to struggle the most with — is loss... loss of friendships, family members, relationships... and losing out on opportunities such as traveling, dating, being further along in my career, and other important events. As someone who is very social and loves to be active and outgoing, not being able to do the things I love with the people I love has been my biggest heartbreak of my ill health.

Editor's Notes About Angela's Healing Journey

- The most important thing anyone can do for themselves is to become their own health and healing advocate. The medical community is looking to treat and fix symptoms, not get to the root cause of the problem, especially when the cases are complicated.
- Perseverance and commitment are essential elements of a healing journey, as the progress is not often linear and you will often face hurdles and setbacks on your way to true healing.
- It often takes multiple modalities of healing to release the layers of trauma that develop over the course of our lives.
- As the wonderful book, The Body Keeps the Score, notes: many people keep unprocessed emotions from past traumas deep in their bodies — resulting in the use of somatics and body movements (including dancing, jumping, hiking, etc.) to release that trauma, resulting in great healing.

Angela's healing journey is an inspiration to many, and she has embraced healing as a profession. She is an Intuitive Reiki Master, Clairvoyant Medium since childhood, and Holistic Health and Wellness Practitioner. Read more from her in Chapter 16: How to Find a Reiki Master/Intuitive Energy Healer.

CHAPTER 25:
Healing Journey Story #6

Ocean: The Deep Waters of Initiation

First Name: George

Age: Generation X

Gender: Male

How/Why You Started on Healing Journey: Fear of death.

Words That Describe Where You are in Your Healing Journey: Unfolding, awareness, non-locality, interdependent, spiritual, meaningful, profound, shadow.

Most Valuable Thing You've Learned on Your Healing Journey: It is through suffering that man becomes like god.

Progress on Your Healing Journey: Spiritual crossroads.

Hardest part of your healing journey: Letting go.

Best Advice to Someone Just Starting Their Healing Journey: Tell everyone you know what happened as soon as possible.... Not for therapy, not for righteousness, because ultimately what happens is you begin making peace and as the days, weeks, even years go by, you run into someone who asks you about your loved one, and then you have to relive their last moments... Again... and...again. This can be an incredibly painful experience! These times cannot be completely avoided but telling everyone, what happened at the time, can dramatically reduce the amount of occurrences.

My Healing Story:

It was January 3, 2011, the day my first child, Ocean, was born. Everyone who has children understands "the ordeal" that is the birth of your first child.

You're, prepping. You go and register at the Babies-R-Us, you get the new stroller, the high chair, you're looking at the latest and greatest new baby equipment — some of which costs thousands of dollars! Of course, you want to buy it all; however, you understand you could never afford it. Friends and family begin showing up at your house in the third trimester with monogrammed bibs, baby clothes, and cloth diapers.

Like other couples embarking on this journey, we were presented with a choice. Would you like to know if it's a boy or a girl? When it came time for the ultrasound we were dying to know; however, the little rascal was camera shy. No matter how much the doctor prodded or pushed the kid was not cooperating. So I guess we're going to have to wait and see.

My wife and I had a lot of fun with it. Making wild predictions: I would say ridiculous things like "What if somehow it's three boys? Triplets? I can feel it's going to be a little boy. I know it! I can feel it!"

My wife's like, "No, it's a girl. I could totally feel it." Looking back, it is such a magical time! I truly wish everyone could experience those particular moments with someone they love.

In the third trimester, on our final trip to the ultrasound, my wife in her swollen radiance, we sought to solve this mystery. However, our kicking, punching, little rascal of a child, remained camera shy. The cheerful doctor's response was something like, I just can't get a good read on it...You know... and finally, he says, "I can't get a good read, but I think it's a girl." The truth is we didn't care. As long as, the baby was healthy, that's all that mattered to me.

As the due date approaches, the anticipation begins to build. You have read all the books, gone to the birthing classes, packed the car for the hospital… waiting for the water to break — on edge, nervous, and now we hurry up and WAIT!

Let me give a stream-of-consciousness idea of how I was feeling as I waited.

My wife, our child, our family, there was no division between the self and the other. There was an absence of anything except my love for her, for my child, and for life itself.

A cosmic beauty decorated the world around me. An indescribable intoxication pours of me, through me. I am mystified.

She was carrying our consciousness, our life. You see, you feel your wife and your child in union, our family together for the first time. Our lives forever woven together. Movements are now visible on the outside of her stomach. "Whoa, that's my baby kicking. I can't wait to hold my child, to look into their eyes, to teach them how to surf, just thinking about how beautiful life is. Hopefully that's how it is for you."

Nine months in, my wife and I go grab some food, and our conversation was as follows:

> *Wife: Hey George, I think something's happening.*
> *Me: Really!?*
> *Wife: Yeah, I think we should go to the doctor. It just kind of feels weird.*
> *Me: Alright… alright… !*

So, we shoot home. We grabbed the bag and put it in the car. Then we shoot down to the hospital and we go to the emergency room.

Me: Are you sure this is ready? I didn't see your water break or anything.
Wife: There's, there is... something happening.

At that moment It was like the whole energy in the room changed a little bit. We are in the emergency room; they bring us upstairs into the receiving area where we had our own little delivery room. We go in there and they call our doctor. My wife is immediately hooked up to the ultrasound.

Our doctor wasn't there yet, so the emergency room staff begin deciphering the bells, whistles, and chaos that is the beginning of a first child being born.

There is something wrong! Time slows to a crawl... slow motion, intense focus, hands clenched slightly shaking the doctor arrived. The sonogram is the machine on which you can see the baby... and monitor the heartbeat... The doctor, I see his eyes narrow, his expression change.

I'm still, like a statue, but my eyes move frantically as I was looking at my wife... the sonogram... the doctor... my wife... the sonogram... the doctor... MY WIFE. The air leaves the room, walls closing in, my world collapsing... time stops. Part of me dies... death. Then without warning, faster than the collapse, a torrential flood of stinging warmth restores me.

At that moment, I notice for the first time in my almost forty years of life that there is a space, nearly imperceptible, less than a second but longer than a lifetime, between stimulus and response.

Wife: (Screaming) Georgie!! What's happening!!!???

Abandonment gives way to helpless surrender.

Doctor: Searching for a pulse, a sign of life, movement. There is nothing.

The silence is deafening.

Doctor: I'm sorry... I'm sorry... I'm sorry. I will give you some time.

Our personal doctor arrives, enters the room; my wife is crying, as am I. The nurse passionately, consolingly, comes over to my wife. The doctor pulls me aside.

Doctor: Mr. Monty. I'm truly sorry, your child has passed. I'm going to give you some more time, but there are some things that are going to begin happening in the next few minutes that we must discuss.
Me: What's going to happen?
Doctor: Mr. Monty, your wife's water is going to break at that time her contractions will begin to increase and we will deliver the baby. You are going to need to start making some hard choices.

Like the sound of an airplane engine coming from a hummingbird, his voice is clear, strong, and yet I find it difficult to comprehend; his words struggle to establish dominance among the angry mob of screaming voices in my head.

Me: What kind of choices are you talking about?
Doctor: Well, when the baby's born, would you like us to incubate the baby? Put the child in the onesie you brought and bring in here for you and your wife to hold? So you can spend some time with them?

Back to my stream of consciousness. Thinking, mind racing, uncharted territory, novelty, unable to thoroughly comprehend, pros and cons. Is this morbid, how do you hold your dead child? I'm FUCKING scared! I don't want to be here! How long have I been here talking to this guy? Where is my wife? We are all alone...I can't save...I... I NEED HER... to get back to her. SHE NEEDS ME! Be strong, wipe your face, no tears. Hold it together... you are a father now!! ACT LIKE IT!!

Me: Thank you Doctor. I need to speak with my wife. We will have some answers for you in a few minutes.
Doctor: Ok.

Fifteen minutes later.

Doctor: We're going to need to start the delivery process when her water breaks; it won't be long after that happens that contractions begin getting closer. Have you thought about holding your child after delivery?

Me: Yes. We have decided that we would rather not.
Doctor: Okay! It's obviously a very difficult decision, and in the event you change your mind let us know.

Almost on cue, my wife's water breaks. Exactly like the doctor said, contractions followed shortly thereafter. Standing bedside by my wife and unborn child, she puts her hand on mine, she looks up, lovingly into my eyes, squeezes my hand with a surprisingly crushing force.

Wife: Start Counting...
Me: Huh... Oh yeah... the Lamaze class.

One... two... three... four... five... breathe,
One... two... three... four... breathe,
One... two... three... breathe,
One... two... PUSH... C'mon Gorgeous — PUSH!
One... PUSH! I can see baby's head —PUSH.

I close my eyes, retreating for a moment into my own cognitive world. I experience and explore that new world I've recently discovered. I take refuge in the eternal moment, between stimulus and response. My thoughts betray me...

Here is more of my internal monologue:

I'm drowning in anguish, assaulted by anxiety, havoc is unleashed on my being, then a magnificent bewilderment momentarily swells to the surface; it's a hierophant. An aleph, a fleeting sensation that leaves me with the slight metallic aftertaste of blood in my mouth... irrationally marvelous.

Immediately I find myself surrounded, consumed, and disoriented. With my senses heightened with adrenaline I hear the primal guttural sound of exhaustion from the woman I love engaged in the ritualistic ceremony, a rite of passage, the bridge from woman to mother, ushering a new life into the world.

Simultaneously I stand strong by her side, ready, willing and able, harboring murderous intent toward her enemies — but ultimately unable to protect her. It is a ceremony. A position alongside her at the ritualistic alter to bear witness to the unthinkable act of our child's death.

Released from the siren's song, I return. I open my eyes. I can see a thick silvery cord, slick with fluid wrapped tightly around our child's neck as he emerges into the light.

Doctor: "It's a BOY!!
Me: It's a BOY!...My son is dead!!! Our child is dead. I knew it was a boy..."
Wife: I want to hold my son!!

These sorts of events tend to bring about an unbreakable bond or tear apart the foundation of a relationship. Lucky for me my incredible wife and I were able to forge the unbreakable bond. It was not without our own individual experience of "The Dark Night of The Soul."

A few years passed by as I tried to make sense of the situation. There were a lot of questions about God, life, love and of course the infamous question "Why Me?" that seemed to be playing on my internal soundtrack, always on repeat.

The Healing Begins

For me the way forward — the path to healing — was shaped liked the Triton of Poseidon, three pointed: psychedelics, nature, and spirituality.

Psychedelics

Psychedelics, particularly psilocybin, allowed me that unique third person perspective that is often without emotion. It's as though you're invited to, or perhaps granted the ability to, focus your awareness not on the surface of the object but on the infinity as seen through the object. As I take a moment to reflect, I think the best way to put it in words is that psychedelics allow for a unified perception.

It was time and a rather large dose, roughly 85mg of 4-AcO-DMT (synthetic mushrooms, similar to the effect from psilocybin), that helped me begin to integrate the trauma.

Alone, in a quiet room, I began to hear a booming voice. It was the first time in my life that I have ever had an audio hallucination. It scared me; I was paralyzed by fear, almost to the point of tears.

The voice asked: “What do you want?”

I said out loud: “I want to understand why. Why me?”

The room collapsed around me and I was transported to my own world, where I was shown a slideshow of ghastly images. Mostly dead children, burned bodies, famine, torture, and of course my son. I begged the voice to stop, but the images kept coming. I could feel pain and sorrow radiate through my body.

Again, I asked the voice to stop.

The booming voice rang out: “I cannot stop. You asked me to show you and there is no turning back.”

After what seemed like hours the images began losing their painful edge.

Realization began to set in that it’s not just me, it’s everyone. Everyone suffers. Lots of people lose children; some people lose their loved ones in ways that are vastly more gruesome than I lost my son.

Some people have their loved ones stolen, murdered, raped or tortured. It sounds crazy but I began to think how lucky, how fortunate I am.

It’s all about perspective: My relationship with my wife was still intact, I was healthy, everyone else in my life was healthy, and I was still able to manage a smile. I had been given a gift!

From this point forward, I was able to recognize my pain, my disappointment, and my fear of death in anyone that I became close with.

It came to me that without suffering, without sacrifice, there can be no salvation and that over time, our greatest tragedies can become our greatest gifts.

Nature

This paradigm-shifting understanding about the relationship between suffering, sacrifice, and salvation led me to look at nature in a new light, a new dimension, with the scales ripped from my eyes.

Our relationship, my wife and I with the Ocean, has always been one of profound respect. So much so that we named our only son after its powerful form. After my son Ocean had died, I spent a lot of time there. In it, on it, or just lying in the sand next to it. In some ways, I feel like the Ocean knew that our son was sacrificed to it... I'm not sure if that can even make any sense to anyone but me.

I honestly feel like the hole in my heart left by my son was filled in, by a force of nature. I like that phrase "A force of nature." I feel like it really captures the idea of what happened to me, what happens to others, and what may be happening to you reading this!

You see, there are some things in life that can never be "learned." They can only be developed inside of you. Only after enough pressure does coal become a diamond, and so too, only after enough pressure can you find the courage, the strength, the faith to become your authentic self.

In the same way the grain of sand on the seashore existed as part of the mountain, so will you become that force of nature that is developing inside you. I've learned that if you're seeking a great teacher, perhaps a waterfall or a battered coastline may have more to say than some of the world's finest institutions.

Nature has become for me, an aleph, a spiritual mirror, where I can see my own fractal image. I am the past, I am the present, I am the future, I exist in all that exists.

Spirituality

Spirituality is like a sixth sense. I think it's important to repeat this idea that, it is not something anyone can ever learn, it can only be developed inside of you, and only after great sacrifice. For me, losing a child is like being granted access to an elite club that no one in the right mind would ever "choose" to join. If you knew the sacrifice that you had to make in order to understand spirituality, I reckon the world would be without a large number of spiritual leaders.

It was that particular "trip" that rekindled my relationship with psychedelics... a path that I have been on ever since. Throughout this healing journey, I've experimented with different protocols, including the Stamets, the Fadiman... even doing daily micro-doses for months at a time.

I don't think there is a magic bullet, a one-size-fits-all, or sure-fire-method that can work for everyone. Like all relationships, my interaction with psychedelics has evolved over the years. However, the one thing that is constant is my use of them.

My usage of plant medicine, while consistent, has varied over the years. After my son's death, once or twice a year seemed to be all I needed in order to begin the integration process. However, over time I began to build a relationship with the medicine, and it became part of me.

Until recently, my most recent pattern of plant medicine has been something along the lines of a large dose, 10-18 grams twice a year, a moderate dose of 5-9 grams every other month, a smaller dose and/or a microdose every 2-3 days for maintenance.

I have followed this regimen pretty closely for the last five years.

Final Thoughts:

In summary, I would just like to say to anyone willing to listen: *No one will ever see things the way you do, ever!*

It's both the most beautiful thing about life and the most tragic. Ultimately, we're all together, alone in unity.

Perhaps, Charles Dickens said it best: "It was the best of times, it was the worst of times."

Editor's Notes About George's Healing Journey

- As unimaginable as it may be for many of us to grasp, George and his family found true healing and insights from the unexpected death of their son, Ocean.
- True healing often requires multiple healing modalities, and as part of a healing journey, you should try any modalities that speak to you.
- While there is a place for every healing modality, there is no question of the power of psychedelic medicines to strip everything away and get to the root issues that need understanding and healing.
- Many people are finding the use of microdosing psychedelics as beneficial for maintaining good mental (and physical) health, reducing levels of anxiety — and without the worry of having a "psychedelic" (hallucinatory) experience.
- We are all part of the natural environment, so it makes sense that deeply immersing ourselves in nature will result in understanding, comprehension, healing.
- One note about dosages. What George calls a large dose, most would call a very deep dose; and what George considers moderate, most would call a heroic dose... but it also depends on the strain and how you measure the psilocybin. As you contemplate your psychedelic experience, be sure to clearly understand dosages.

George is a husband and father, as well as a seeker of knowledge and insights. He is owner of TrueLife Media, an amazing podcaster, and a communication specialist. Learn more at his website: https://truelife.transistor.fm/

CHAPTER 26:
Healing Journey Story #7

A Healing Story of the Forest and the Dragonflies

First Name: Kat

Age: Millennial

Gender: Female

How/Why You Started on Healing Journey: My own body spoke loudly and clearly to let me know the lifestyle I adopted was not supportive for my health and well-being.

Words That Describe Where You are in Your Healing Journey: Currently healed and well, using the tools I have gathered on the way to bring myself back to harmony with (my inner) nature again whenever needed.

Most Valuable Thing You've Learned on Your Healing Journey: That everything is relational, including our relationship with the rest of nature and the nature that we are. That all things of value grow from inner peace.

Progress on Your Healing Journey: My body and mind are fully healed and connected, with no medications involved.

Hardest Part of Your Healing Journey: Moments when it was necessary to accept what is, rather than resisting it. Having patience and trust.

Best Advice to Someone Just Starting Their Healing Journey: A restful nature moment each day keeps the doctor away.

My Healing Story:

This is a story of a little girl who loved nothing more than spending entire summer days sitting up in the branches of an old willow tree that she called her 'office.' A story of getting lost and disconnected from nature. A story of bumps in the road where the body worked as a messenger informing about the need for radical change of direction. A story about rediscovering nature as a portal to reconnection, joy, and healing.

My name is Kat Novotna and I'm a Forest Therapy Guide, the originator of EcoNIDRA, mentor in presence and self-care and mom of one little Viking. Nature connection work is my mission, passion, and my calling. It is completely aligned with my heart and the medicines or gifts that Mother Nature wants me to use and share with others and be of service to Her. It is work that supports my own physical, mental, and emotional health, and gives me energy rather than depleting myself. And it wasn't always like that, nor is this story complete now. It is a healing story of the *Forest and the Dragonflies*.

The child who was living completely in the present moment and feeling one with nature eventually went to school. In school, they taught me to sit at a desk, to do my homework, to achieve goals and have high standards. They taught me to not move or sing unless it was a music or sports class, and to do my best to get the best grades — so to be acknowledged and loved by my teachers, parents, and eventually, and especially, myself.

I was a good girl and adopted the requirements of the modern society as if they were my own. I studied even harder, got even better grades, learned to speak multiple languages, started my own business... and ultimately spent 14 to 16 hours a day facing a computer screen in an attempt to get all the work done.

After twenty years of disembodiment cultivated at desks, I was not able to hear or respect the signals of my own body: the fatigue, the irritability; the sugar and coffee addiction; the bloating, tired, red, and itchy eyes. The show must go on, the next deadline was getting closer, and every next task was a yes.

The signals from my body that were gentle and mild at first, became louder: my body had to speak loudly and clearly in order to get any attention at all, and so it did. My eyes got inflamed and the inflammation of both eyes became a very painful and chronic issue to the point where I couldn't even keep my eyes open for longer than two seconds. I had to stop typing, reading, and checking my emails; I had to stop working. *I had to STOP the madness.*

No medication, antibiotics, eye drops, or air moisturizers were able to heal the chronical inflammation –and so I spent a few months in despair, sitting in a chair, listening to audio books. Since air in indoor spaces is shared with others, as well as the constant air conditioning, these were environments that were unbearable for my eyes, and since I could not work anyway, I started to take gentle, careful, and slow walks in the forest.

These walks were actually more of a sit spot that allowed me to keep my eyes closed most of the time. I discovered that the forest sounds calmed me and the despair wasn't as overwhelming as it was in other environments. I realized that the forest air was the only air that was nice and gentle for my hurting and inflamed eyes.

Once I could keep my eyes open for longer, I noticed that all the green and brown shades of nature, as well as the relief to my eyes, mind, and emotions. The slow pace was something completely new for someone who was used to efficiently making use of every single minute of the day.

The forest became my sanctuary and my daily bread, and I adopted the slow pace of trees and leaves in the wind. Something had changed in me, and slowly but surely, my eyes were healing. Believe it or not, my eyes that used to be rather blue turned green too.

Slowly, I learned my lesson about what conditions my body needed to live in, and about that my natural habitat is nature. I realized my old coffee-run, stress-hormones-based, sugar-addicted, and tiring lifestyle was not what I was born for.

I connected to the stillness of nature and rediscovered myself, my own nature.

Shortly after that, I walked into a bookstore and stumbled upon a book with a beautiful tree drawing on the front cover and a title that grabbed my attention: *Shinrin-yoku — Forest Bathing.* I couldn't resist getting it and read the complete book the same night. Written by the Japanese scientist Dr. Qing Li, the book was my introduction to something that would change my life completely — the art of forest bathing.

I learned about scientific research backing up what I experienced in the forest, and that one could actually train to become a Forest Bathing guide. I immediately signed up for a training with the international Association of Nature and Forest Therapy (ANFT). Within two weeks, I was on my way to Slovenia, the nearest training in 2018, to become a guide. Arriving to the training location, I was full of excitement and curiosity: Whom would I meet there? Will I land in a group of Japanese scientists? Foresters? Witches...? Is this really something for me? Will they require me to have a lot of factual knowledge about trees that I don't have?

Within two days I felt completely reassured that I was exactly on the right track, with exactly the right people. I felt something that I now call a *love attack* — a strong heart-felt realization that following my intuition to become a Forest Therapy guide was the most important step in my life. Years after, it still feels that way. I strongly felt that it is my mission to spread this deep nature connection that I cultivated with the world.

After being certified as a Forest Therapy guide, I started to guide many people on forest therapy walks and kept deepening my awe and sense of wonder about what the forest can do for humans when we allow it to be the therapist, and what can arise when humans remember their relationship with nature deeply written in their DNA. I remembered the little girl sitting up in her willow tree office, and with a smile on my face and healthy eyesight, I went on spreading the magic as a Forest Therapy guide and trainer of guides with the ANFT.

The amazing thing about the way nature can heal us if we are rested enough to receive it is that it does not seem to only treat one condition like typical medications do. Yes, my eyes healed, but then my digestion and my sleep improved, my sugar addiction was gone, my moods stabilized, and the relationship with my own body changed for the better.

Most importantly, with the forest therapy, I reconnected with my heart, with the true essence of who or what I am, outside

the daily busyness and the pressures of what we call the modern lifestyle.

But it would be too idealistic to think that there is only beauty, bliss, and joy in nature. Of course, nothing is black or white, and there are also things to be aware of when you spend a lot of time in wild nature. One of them are ticks — ticks that live in many climates and carry diseases.

After many delicious and happy years spent in forests, among mosses and grasses that I would never want to miss, one day I got diagnosed with Lyme disease.

The incredibly intelligent Lyme bacteria in my body brought me days when I could live my life for no longer than two hours a day. For the rest of the time, I was too fatigued to even stay awake. Is this chronic fatigue? Is this how my life was going to look like now? Both the doctors and the internet said it might be the case.

More Forest Healing:

As a Forest Therapy guide and someone who had remembered and cultivated a deep connection and respect for all nature — including my own body — I knew the way for me to go was by stimulating my own immune system to allow the body to heal. The best way to do this would be to go into my beloved forest and let the phytoncides emitted by trees do their work on the Natural Killer cells of my body's own immune system. But how do you do this when you can barely even walk?

I remembered something. It was a feeling. The feeling of waking up on a meadow on one beautiful warm summer day back in 2015. I was lying on my back after a yoga Nidra session at a

Yoga Festival on one of the Dutch islands in the beautiful grassy sand dunes near the ocean. It was a feeling of total bliss, being completely relaxed and energized at the same time, feeling fully alive and in deep love with all the nature beings surrounding me on that meadow.

Remembering this experience, I started practicing yoga Nidra while laying on my back in the Shavasana pose at home every day. What happened within a couple of weeks was almost a miracle — not only was I able to stay awake again, I gained all my energy back — and some more — and some profound soul healing happened for me exactly where it needed to happen.

I felt refreshed and nourished like never before. I was symptom and pain-free, and with a sense of deep inner peace and deeper awareness. I started to study yoga Nidra and became a certified yoga Nidra teacher.

At that stage, the new vital energy that I cultivated allowed me to do solo walks in the forest again, where I had beautiful encounters with dragonflies — the ancient beings that have been on planet Earth for millions of years. The colors, the elegance of their flight, the sound, the feeling of vibrant presence when they would stop right in front of me and I came to look at them eye to eye...

Dragonflies and damselflies kept coming back to me, flying around in circles, and sitting on my body so often that I decided to look up the symbolism of dragonflies as they were known to ancient cultures and civilizations. As it turned out, in ancient times, dragonflies were considered beings that were able to travel between different dimensions. They were also believed to be connected to human beings and willing to guide them through different dimensions of perception and consciousness.

These fascinating beings of nature inspired me to create the practice of Econidra, and to train certified Econidra teachers, guides who'd be like dragonflies: guiding others through different dimensions of consciousness, reconnecting people and the Earth. Yoga Nidra is able to do that and as a Forest Therapy guide, I feel the relation with nature is in every single atom of our beings, so it made perfect sense to me to create a blend of both worlds that would help people to relax and reconnect with nature, with themselves and with others, even if they cannot spend hours and hours in nature.

Amazing that one hungry tick, as well as the super-intelligent Lyme bacteria, ultimately brought me to even deeper nature connection, thankfulness for every single day that I have the vital energy to do what I want to do, and, even created a new practice that, like Forest Bathing, is now helping thousands of people to heal, reconnect with nature, with their body and with themselves, and to get energized and rested enough to achieve whatever their heart desires.

As of today, I'm very grateful for the deep nature connection that I rediscovered and that brought back that little girl sitting up in the willow tree. I'm grateful for my eyes that at some point didn't give me another choice but to go out into the forest and change my lifestyle completely.

I'm grateful to the Lyme bacteria that for a moment paralyzed me allowed me to rise like a (dragonfly) phoenix from the ashes of chronic fatigue.

Key insight:

Nature, and the practices of Forest Bathing and Econidra, help us relax and reconnect so that we can heal and get inspired.

As someone who has quite recently experienced motherhood for the first time, I can say these practices have immensely helped me through everything related to a problematic pregnancy — preparation for giving birth, post-partum recovery, lack of sleep, etc.

Deep nature connection, Forest Bathing, and Econidra are my one apple a day that not only keeps the doctor away, but also allows me to enjoy this precious period with vital energy, loving relationships, and high levels of presence and consciousness most of the time.

The forest has our back, and I truly believe that nature-connected and well-rested people can change the world.

Editor's Notes About Kat's Healing Journey

- Living apart from nature is truly unnatural for us — as well as unhealthy. You can still live in a city or town and experience nature, but the key is taking the time to truly commune and experience nature... enjoying time resting, walking, playing, and dancing in nature.
- All forest bathers stress the healing benefits of phytoncides, but what are they? Phytoncides are volatile organic compounds (VOCs) — tree essential oils — that have many medicinal properties, including regulating the nervous system and reducing blood glucose levels, as well as anti-inflammatory and mood-enhancing effects.
- Natural killer cells (NK cells) are white blood cells that destroy infected and diseased cells, like cancer cells; a 2-hour walk in the forest increases NK cell activity that can last for days.
- Lyme disease is an ugly and debilitating condition — physical pain, fatigue, and brain fog are just some of the worst effects. Early detection is key. Side note: Almost ALL ticks carry some type of disease, so it is extremely important to check yourself after time spent outdoors in the spring and summer.

Kat is a Forest Therapy Guide, founder of EcoNIDRA™ and Way Back Home, Mentor in Presence & Self-Care, Kintsugi artist, and mom of one little Viking. Her passion and mission are to help people reconnect with nature, with themselves and with others. Learn more here: www.waybackhome.info

CHAPTER 27:
Healing Journey Story #8

I Needed to Heal But Didn't Know It at the Time

First Name: Tristan

Age: Millennial

Gender: Male

How/Why You Started on Healing Journey: By accident! It all started through the power of breathing. My now wife bought me a breathwork session as a surprise birthday present. At the time, I was working in finance in a large corporation and the work I'd done on myself was all focused on developing myself to be more successful in my career.

Words That Describe Where You are in Your Healing Journey: I'm 7 years into a lifelong journey of healing, learning, and growing. Breathwork has been an amazing tool for me, and has brought so much more natural energy and vitality into my life, from a physiological perspective, but it has also helped me from a psychological perspective. Working with some amazing mentors, in combination with breathwork, has allowed me to uncover and heal many blind spots and limiting beliefs, which were draining my energy, particularly in moments of pressure or stress.

Most Valuable Thing You've Learned on Your Healing Journey: Connection to myself and to others. For most of my life, I'd felt disconnected, and this was because I wasn't being my authentic self. For more than 30 years, I'd created an identity based on decisions I made as a child... including my personality (people-pleasing because I lost all my close friends as a young teenager), career (I became a banker because I never wanted the money issues I experienced as a child) and never crying (because I was told as a child that crying is for girls).

Progress on Your Healing Journey: Breathwork and inner work has helped me to heal things from my past that were holding me back in ways I never realized. It's helped me unlock new levels of emotional intelligence, which I believe is a superpower for people in leadership roles. I see the inner work as being like peeling back layers of an onion; the work continues and as I free myself from my limiting beliefs and self-destructive thought patterns, life becomes easier and I become happier.

Hardest Part of Your Healing Journey: Forgiveness. Not of other people, but of myself. I've always been a high-achiever, and my own biggest critic.

Best Advice to Someone Just Starting Their Healing Journey: Find what works for you. For me, it was the breath. But there are so many amazing tools and healing modalities out there.

My Healing Story:

I can see these three things now as childhood traumas, but at the time, it was simply about living my life.

- *I lost all my close friends as a young teenager:* as is often the case, during my adolescent years, the most important thing to me was belonging and being connected with my friendship group. In my mid-teens I started to drift from the group. With the benefit of hindsight, being cut from the group was positive; we had very different values, beliefs, interests, and journeys to go on. At the time I was heartbroken and felt lost, alone and worthless. I spent the next year drifting on the edge of different friendship groups, which felt really tough.

I adapted my personality to become as likable and amenable as possible as a winning formula for making friends. This started to work, but as I grew older I would find myself feeling drained from the people-pleasing. Through healing I learned how empowering it is to speak your truth and that those truly connected to you will love and respect you for your genuine perspectives.

- I *never wanted the money issues I experienced as a child:* I grew up in a working-class family and my lovely parents did an amazing job, but as a young couple with 3 children, things were often tough financially. This left an unconscious imprint that money is hard to come by and there often isn't enough to go round.

These limiting beliefs had a positive consequence in making me determined to succeed in my career and create abundance for myself and my family. The downside is that I unconsciously attached a huge part of my identity and self-worth to success in my career, including success with promotions; but, progression was never enough to create lasting fulfillment and happiness.

- *Told as a child that crying is for girls:* as a sensitive and emotional boy growing up in northern England, I was told by family members, teachers, sports coaches, and strangers that crying is not something that boys do.

I quickly learned to suppress my emotions, and I left that door relatively locked until my first breathwork session.

Before I started my healing journey, I had a successful career and a winning formula that involved having a positive mindset, focusing on goals for the future, and being highly disciplined. I attended courses, attended seminars, and read books on personal development, *but my biggest blind spot was I didn't see that I needed to heal.*

Just to add more pressure, on top of work, I was also attending business school in the evenings, studying for my MBA.

On the outside, I appeared to have it all together. I would even try to convince myself of this, but I realized through my healing journey that my drive was often coming from a place of lack. Lack of deep self-confidence, trust, and identity. I would use my success and achievements to hide how I really felt deep down.

I hated talking about challenging times or problems from the past. It left me feeling worse, so I wouldn't go there. Focusing on the future and positive situations felt better, but I always felt a deep sense of disconnection from myself and from others. I failed to see the two things could be linked.

At some point, I realized I was experiencing pretty severe depression, exhaustion, and anxiety.

I went to the doctor. He suggested I take a break and start medication. I realized doctors are trained to diagnose symptoms, not the underlying cause.

I needed to find my own solution.

I started to see the scientific links between energy, mood, emotions, nutrition, gut health, psychology, and the way we breathe.

The Healing Begins

Breathwork changed everything for me.

I discovered energy, power, and happiness in facing into the darkest parts of myself that I'd tried to hide from everyone (including myself). I've always hated talking about my pain and problems — it just made me feel worse.

Combining the somatic healing of the breath, with understanding my life journey and cognitive development and how thought patterns from my childhood continued to play out in my subconscious as an adult, gave me a completely *different perspective*... and new power and energy.

After my first rebirthing breathwork session, I cried for the first time in more than a decade. To be perfectly honest, if I'd known this would happen, I probably wouldn't have done it.

But after the session, I felt like a huge emotional weight had been lifted from my shoulders. I don't know why I cried; the breath worker explained to me that we store feelings and emotions in the cellular memory of our body and by breathing we can release and heal. The logical part of my brain questioned this, but I couldn't deny how good it felt, which allowed me to go deeper and deeper.

As I progressed with my healing journey, I realized that I'd been living my life only allowing myself to feel a very narrow set of emotions. Being a man, I'd suppressed the more "feminine" emotions associated with crying.

Having a professional career, I'd also denied myself the most "masculine" emotions such as anger. I felt these emotions didn't serve me.

What I'd missed was that experiencing the full spectrum of emotions is part of the beautiful experience of being a human and that this was creating the deep sense of disconnection.

Through the practice of breathwork, I was able to go deep really quickly. It helped me to reconnect with my body and my emotions, and I found a deeper sense of happiness from this place.

The really surprising thing was that I also started to feel deeper connections with other people as well.

I'd been a leader from quite a young age. At 26, I managed a team of nearly 200 people but my manager at the time told me that I needed to work on my emotional intelligence. My solution to this was to read books on EQ, which gave me some knowledge that I brought to my role. But I was always in my mind, thinking about the next question to ask my team and was never truly present. This left me feeling drained.

As I started connecting with myself and healing, I found my emotional intelligence increased. I found I was able to pick up on subtle queues from people about how they were really feeling and I started to trust my intuition more and more, which allowed me to be really present and to listen to people.

When I started being the passionate, emotional, fully expressed man that I felt I'd always been deep down, I felt more energy in my life and I started to create more meaningful connections to other people. As I explored and revealed my own true identity, passions and purpose, I was able to make decisions like my career, colleagues and friends from a place that was much more aligned with my purpose.

It's a journey, which I'm really enjoying. I'm not any kind of healing guru. I love sharing the things that have worked for me, and work for my clients, and I learn just as much from each person I work with, which is also part of my own healing journey.

Why I love breathwork so much:

Using breathing techniques showed me the power of expressing your emotions, even the unpleasant ones. I experienced a spiritual and emotional weight being lifted from my shoulders by releasing my emotions. The best thing for me was that I didn't have to revisit or discuss the painful or sad moments in my life to do this, I just had to breathe.

Final Thoughts:

My healing journey has given me what I wanted — greater tools and success with my work, but it also gave me so much more. This connection with others also transferred into my personal life, with my partner, my friends, and my family.

Last Words:

We are all unique — and if you're interested in understanding if there could be healing in the breath for you, I'd be happy to talk or guide you through a session to see if breathing resonates.

Editor's Notes About Tristan's Healing Journey

- One of the saddest common denominators across men of a certain age is that many of us were told as boys that crying was for girls, sissies, babies. From that message, we learn that suppressing our emotions is the safest route.
- One of the dirty little secrets that many have known for years is that trauma is often a powerful force that drives us to succeed (so that we don't have the time to revisit the past).
- While the focus of healing is using whatever modalities that best resonate with you, it's rare that one modality is powerful enough to power a healing journey... but it's always important to lean into the healing.
- Breathwork is the easiest and cheapest healing modality; it takes no special equipment, no big investments — except an investment in time and a commitment to healing.

Tristan coaches people to master their breath and energy... from tired and stressed to energized and in flow... dissolving stress and pressure. Learn more at his website: www.tristanrushworth.com

CHAPTER 28:
Healing Journey Story #9

Microdosing for Love

Name: Megan

Age: Generation Z

Gender: Female

How/Why You Started on Healing Journey: Healing anxiety and depression.

Words That Describe Where You are in Your Healing Journey: Content and optimistic.

Most Valuable Thing You've Learned on Your Healing Journey: If you are struggling with love, look at inner child wounds from family.

Progress on Your Healing Journey: Better emotional regulation, challenging black and white thinking, more presence.

Hardest Part of Your Healing Journey: Learning to let go.

Best Advice to Someone Just Starting Their Healing Journey: Start with the modality you are most interested in.

My Background

My name is Megan and I am 26 years old. I currently live in Chicago and am originally from the western suburbs. I grew up in a upper-middle class, Irish Catholic household, which means my sisters and I were all competitive high achievers in school and sports.

Our parents and community held excellence as the baseline for achievement, so needless to say that from a young age, I put a lot of pressure on myself to be the best in all aspects of life.

This also led to burn-out by the time I hit college.

Studying mechanical engineering at a top 20 university was hard to be proud of when I felt so burned out with life. There was a noticeable shift in my mental health. I had always been an anxious kid growing up, struggling with social anxiety and performance anxiety. These were highly normalized in my community, so I didn't think much of my anxiety other than it was something that felt annoying and made me feel inferior to others.

However, in college, I started feeling even more anxious, with the pressures of academic excellence kicked up higher, and for the first time in my life, *I was dealing with depression crashes.*

I didn't know what to do other than brute force my way through undergrad. It was here that I started to question who I was, what was my purpose, and how to feel good in my skin, which was the ultimate start to my healing journey.

From college, I started looking to food as medicine to help with the stress-related hormonal imbalances, and after graduating, I started seeing a therapist to help with my mental health. I was lucky that my therapist was also a yoga therapist, so she was more holistic in her practice and introduced me to meditation.

Mediation has been the ULTIMATE game changer and continues to be my favorite modality for healing.

My hormonal imbalances started to regulate even more so with adding this to my clean diet changes, and my cycle started coming back after 4 years of no menstruation. I felt more at ease; I felt like I could breathe again.

From therapy, I went on to pursue my yoga teaching training certification, Reiki certification, and took a deep dive into all the healing modalities I could study. From yoga and Reiki came EMDR therapy and astrology... and I started feeling more lit up and aligned with myself.

I had a newfound wonder and childlike joy that I hadn't felt in a long time.

Then, in 2021, I started coming across podcasts and documentaries on psychedelics for healing.

My microdosing journey

And now for the fun (yet still challenging!) part of my healing journey. I had listened to quite a few podcasts on psychedelics for most of 2021, and at the end of the year, I discovered a local Meetup group led by Matt Simpson that discussed microdosing. I was intrigued, went to the next group meeting, and I was so thrilled to know there were other people like me who were either eager enthusiasts or current microdosers wanting to learn from others.

I learned about the benefits of microdosing, who is a good fit to try microdosing, and how it differs from classic peak experiences. I especially loved learning about the concept of neural plasticity, that your brain can rewire old neural pathways to form more positive beliefs about yourself and the world. I decided that at some point, I would set aside time for myself to try microdosing to see what benefits it had on me versus the countless other modalities I had tried.

A few months went by. I had just gotten out of a short-term relationship with a woman, and I was feeling really low. I had struggled a lot with anxious attachment in this relationship, and I knew that there was a deeper wound to heal so I could feel more stable and aligned in my next love connection. So I figured, "Well let's see how microdosing can help with my confidence in dating."

I still remember my first day taking a psilocybin microdose. I was on a run on an unseasonably warm February in Chicago, and I felt AMAZING! I was running with my arms wide open, taking in the fresh air and feeling so alive. I knew from that day that microdosing would be a good fit for me, and I was excited to see what benefits it would bring to me on both my conscious and subconscious mind.

My first experience microdosing was with the Fadiman protocol. This entailed taking a 0.07 — 0.1 gram microdose of psilocybin every 3 days. On one day, off two days in microdose speak. I enjoyed this protocol because it was fairly low maintenance, yet powerful. Even on off days, I still felt slightly more energized and focused than my usual baseline.

Outside of improved energy levels, I noticed more creativity in my day to day. I was less bogged down by work problems but rather more excited to get creative with solutions. This even translated into more creativity in my wardrobe, feeling more interested in my own self-expression through fashion. Overall, the boosts of energy and creativity led to greater self-confidence. I had yet to bridge the gap to confidence in love though, so I decided to reach out to Matt Simpson to be my microdosing coach as I focused on calling in love.

I worked with Matt for 8 weeks during the spring and early summer of 2022. He had me follow the Stamets Stack protocol this time around, which involved 0.07-0.1 gram psilocybin doses 5 days a week: 5 days on, 2 off. In addition to the psilocybin, the Stamets Stack involved adding Niacin (vitamin B3) and Lion's Mane mushroom, taking all three ingredients together in one capsule.

With the more frequent dosing and the added functional ingredients, the Stamets Stack kicked it up a notch, and the effects were more prominent. I noticed more energy and focus, which was especially helpful since I was wanting to go deep on what blocks I may have in love and relationships.

As you can tell from me mentioning that my last partner was a woman, I identify as a queer person. This was a part of my identity I greatly struggled with up until my mid-twenties. I never wanted anyone to know that I may be queer, so as a result, I dimmed my light a lot in my teens and college years. I tried to avoid my queer identity like the plague, but once I started therapy after college, I started coming to terms with who I am and experiencing more self-love and acceptance.

I put myself out there on the dating apps, came out to my friends and family, and started owning my identity more and more each day. By the time I started microdosing with Matt, I considered myself pretty comfortable with my queer identity. I had gone to Pride events and was starting to form my queer community in Chicago, but I knew that there was still some internalized homophobia that was plaguing my subconscious.

Setting my intention around calling in a female romantic partner was the direction my subconscious needed to rewire old neural pathways preventing my aligned love from coming through. And the psilocybin microdosing was the perfect tool to enhance my neural plasticity.

For the next 8 weeks, I followed the Stamets stack protocol, adjusted dosage sizes as needed, and talked with Matt once a week to check in on my progress. Matt also had me doing Wim Hof breathing for 10 minutes every morning to help enhance the mood benefits with microdosing. I loved having that routine every morning on top of my morning meditations, and during the week, Matt would give me journal prompts to probe at what beliefs could be blocking my connection to love.

Inner child work was the theme of those 8 weeks! If I learned anything from this work, it's that your relationship to your primary caretakers sets the foundation for your love patterns going forward. And for me, I had a complicated relationship with my dad, especially when it came to my queerness. Coming out to him and my mom was not easy; it was met with more questioning who I was than acceptance of me.

While things have gotten easier as time has gone on, especially with my mom, there has become a distance between me and my dad when it comes to our current relationship. It feels like "don't ask, don't tell," which in a way feels better than outright rudeness.

Even outside of queerness, I have routinely felt not enough in my dad's eyes, always needing to push for more and achieve more. Get the higher grade, get into the best school possible, make the most money. But even when I would achieve a high grade or perform well in a sport, it never was enough to make him feel happy. Hello perfectionism and people-pleasing roots.

As you can read, there is a core wound of wishing to be loved and accepted fully as I am by my dad, and this block has translated to blocks in love.

How could I call in my aligned partner when deep down, I was holding onto old limiting beliefs around being "enough" from my dad? How could I feel deserving of being loved fully if I didn't feel that way with my parent?

To heal this wound, I worked on reparenting myself to feel whole in all that I am. Journaling, deep meditations and reframing old memories were all a part of this inner child healing. The degree in which I went in to heal inner child wounds associated with my dad was the degree I was able to shine out as more confident and radiant.

Doing this heavy inner healing was made a bit easier with microdosing; I felt I had the bandwidth to go in and face these wounds without getting sucked into the shadows. So yes, my microdosing journey went deep, and my subconscious was put to work to rewire limiting beliefs around worth and my queerness so I could call in my aligned partner.

Love coming through

After the 8 weeks with Matt, I noticed a huge shift in my dating. At that point, I had gotten out of another short-term relationship with someone, and I yet again felt really low about it. I wasn't afraid to feel the lowness, and I had more trust that I would get back to feeling more regulated and whole again.

Dating for the rest of the summer became A LOT more frequent! I had women coming up to me at bars and asking me out, which had NEVER happened before. The women I dated at the time were quality people, who checked off a lot on my list as far as partner traits. I had fun with dating and felt more go with the flow.

What is funny is in early August, I actually decided to put a pause on dating. At that point, I had a busy summer, I dated a lot of women, and I now wanted to redirect my attention to other aspects of my life, trusting that my partner would come through when she (or they) and I were both ready.

I know everyone says "love happens when you least expect it" but I secretly thought people that said that weren't "trying hard enough" in love. Don't worry, I have since connected the dots with my conditioning on work and worth and don't think this way anymore. ☺

About 3 weeks after pausing the dating apps, I met my now partner. We met at my favorite bar in Chicago during a friend's birthday, and the rest was history. I had never felt so safe yet excited with someone. Right off the bat, they checked off a lot of my list: passionate, good sense of humor, confident, goal-oriented, caring deeply about friends and family, and of course incredibly beautiful.

Meeting someone like this in the past used to trigger my anxious attachment. I would become worried if I was enough for them, if they would drop off unexpectedly, if I was worthy of their love in the end. Not surprisingly, all the inner work I had done with microdosing paid off, and I had a feeling of ease and confidence with Eva, like I could be my full self without fear of judgment.

I took my time with getting to know Eva, letting our connection play out and eventually naturally evolve into our current relationship. I had and have never felt like this with someone before; so seen and so safe, so loved and embraced for all that I am. I feel so lucky that in a relatively short time, I was able to do the inner work and meet someone that I love and care about so deeply.

Life since microdosing

Since microdosing (and having met my partner!), I have continued my exploration of healing modalities. I have become a fan of kundalini yoga in the mornings, different forms of breathwork, and continuing to meditate daily. My confidence in love has translated to more confidence in other aspects of my life, and

I am now the host of a health and wellness podcast called the Brave Psychonaut!

The gift of microdosing is added courage to doing the inner shadow work... adding jet fuel to the intention setting. The degree you go in is the degree you shine out, as Matt Simpson likes to say, so if you are finding yourself stuck on an issue, struggling to find your way through a block, then I highly recommend looking into microdosing.

If I had to give any advice for someone interested, I would say allow yourself to play around with dosing. I found for myself "less is more", so I actually wound up only needing 0.05 grams for microdosing on the Stamets Stack protocol vs 0.07-0.1 grams. Take this process at a pace that is manageable for you, because this is your healing journey after all! And if you find that microdosing doesn't jive with you, then don't be afraid to let go and move on to your more aligned healing modality.

I am so grateful to have experienced this healing modality and seen positive results. I really believe that the microdosing in combination with morning breathwork, meditation, and journaling was my remedy for healing. As big triggers come up in life, as new challenges arise, I feel confident knowing I have my healing toolkit in my back pocket.

Editor's Notes About Megan's Story

- The key to any healing journey is experimenting and finding the healing modalities that work best for you. And as Megan demonstrates, be open to new modalities that arise.
- As with Megan's experience, many high-achieving people are succeeding through the trauma, but there comes a time when that trauma either brings things crashing down or the person begins a healing journey.
- Childhood trauma — and in this case that trauma was "acceptance" and "conditional" love based on performance, not based on the person — is fairly common in our society. With this type of trauma, people can spend their whole lives trying to live up to an image of themselves they can never achieve.
- Microdosing psychedelics (especially psilocybin) is a healing modality getting a lot of buzz because of the MANY anecdotal stories of healing, including Megan's inner child work. These substances are considered by many as powerful tools for healing — but remember that all healing journeys take work and a commitment to integrating the healing into your life.

CHAPTER 29:
Healing Journey Story #10

I Didn't Need a Healing Journey — Until I Did!

First Name: Me'Shell

Age: Generation X

Gender: Female

How/Why You Started on Healing Journey: For the longest time, I thought everything was okay; not perfect, but okay. One day I woke up and didn't recognize myself. I was lost.

Words That Describe Where You are in Your Healing Journey: A work in progress; still working hard on the self-love part.

Most Valuable Thing You've Learned on Your Healing Journey: Two things. First, that probably everyone needs to be on a healing journey. Second, that there are truly beautiful-hearted people in this world who simply want to see people heal.

Progress on Your Healing Journey: I have made massive strides since my journey began, but I have more to unpack and try to understand and grow.

Hardest Part of Your Healing Journey: It's going to sound a bit pathetic, but the hardest part was how long it took to finally recognize I needed to be on a healing journey.

Best Advice to Someone Just Starting Their Healing Journey: Please do it even if you don't think you need one! Just the benefit of rediscovering the joy of my inner child is enough to warrant healing, but there are so many other benefits as well, including love. Take that first step!

My Healing Story:

I'm a product of the inner city. I love the pace, the ease of getting around, and I've never left it. I mean, I am in a better place now than when I was growing up. Back then, I guess you could say I grew up in the ghetto. I don't think I necessarily saw it that way as a kid, but looking back I see that the high-rises of my complex were kind of depressing.

I thought I escaped unscathed from my childhood. I remember hard times, fighting between my parents, and lots of times when we struggled to put food on the table. But there were also happy times with friends, birthday parties, and playgrounds. I do have what I call my fuzzy years, some periods where I really can't recall much about my life, but I thought that was pretty typical of everyone.

I grew up with one other sibling, a brother. He got involved with some bad influences in his teens, which added a lot of fears and tension. He actually got badly hurt in some gang fight, but now as an adult, he is thriving. No issues. We aren't close or anything, but we don't hate each other either. Just different people; always have been.

Me? I struggled in school... mostly. I don't know if it was attention deficit disorder, lazy brain, or maybe trauma that caused me to not like school, to act up in school. I just never got hooked on school.

Otherwise, it was just a march through childhood and adolescence, keeping my head down (mostly), and doing my best not to mess up in ALL things, especially with my brother's gang and drug issues. I also had a few issues with puberty (boobs, my cycle, weight gain, etc.), but nothing really bad or anything that I can remember.

As a young adult, I sure had my struggles, but I also had lots of fun. I was a party girl and loved going out clubbing with my girlfriends... drinking and dancing. A lot of drinking, but never to a dangerous level, like blacking out. *(I did do some party drugs, but I was wary and careful because of my brother.)*

And as an X'er, I have to admit I kind of loved fitting into the stereotype — that no one really got me, got my generation... especially one who grew up where and how I did. It was a badge of honor I wore... kind of like, *don't mess with me.*

And, you know? I did all the things we're supposed to do as adults... I found a job, worked hard, and eventually moved into my own apartment in the city. I had friends, both from work and my neighborhood. I visited my folks occasionally.

Life seemed okay. I worked, came home, watched DVDs or television, and went to bed. I had some fun times on weekends and vacations with friends. Life was good, right? And the years just went by.

I lived that way, alone, for about 20 years. I thought I was content. I had a job, an apartment, and made decent money. I ate pretty badly, never exercised, but I was in generally good health. I took vacations and thought things were good.

I also had my share of dates during those years, but nothing ever substantial, and I really never kept in touch with any of those people. Looking back now, I can clearly see the issue, but during those years, I just felt like I was doing things everyone does at my age.

The Healing Begins

About five years ago, I met the most magical person, and I had my first real relationship. I was in love, I thought. It lasted about a year; a year of so many ups and downs. When it ended, it truly felt like my heart was torn in two.

I was *really* lost for the first time in my life. I didn't feel as though I knew myself. I didn't know what was wrong with me and why I was so alone. I felt isolated and alone for the first time. It was weird, scary, and I thought maybe I was losing my mind; I definitely knew I had lost my heart.

A friend from work told me about a meditation retreat she was thinking about attending. I had no interest at first; meditating looked and sounded like a big waste of time. But as the time drew closer and my feelings of loneliness grew, I took her up on the offer, really, just so I could be part of something.

I just sensed that I needed to try something to get unstuck, meet new people, and find a way to fix my broken heart.

The first day of the retreat changed my life forever and put me on a healing journey, though again, I was not aware of the term nor the need for one. That first day, after some initial nervousness and anxiety (and a lot of doubt), during the third meditation session of the day — outside on this flagstone patio — I discovered a voice deep within me that told me I was worthy of love.

Worthy of love? Of course, I was worthy of love... or was I?

I fought the concept of healing, trauma, abuse. I never experienced any of these things!! Or did I? And what about my parents and their parents? Could trauma truly be passed down from one generation to the next? I know I was never a fan of my parent's parenting, but I knew many of my schoolmates had it MUCH worse than I did.

Still. That one retreat, that I only knew about because of a coworker (who I was not even that close to), was the beginning of a journey I am still on today. I think of it more as a journey of rediscovery than healing, but I have found deep pockets of hurt within me that I never knew existed.

That one retreat also led me on a spiritual journey. The more I combined meditation with breathwork, the deeper I got into myself, learning new things — both good and bad. Through it all, though, I felt a connection to a higher power that I had never experienced. My upbringing had been mostly agnostic.

The following year, I found another retreat, this one more focused on nature and a totally new term to me: forest bathing. This retreat combined meditation and breathwork with long periods of time in a lush forest. I left this retreat with still greater understanding of myself and my place in the world.

Even with this increased awareness, I still felt there were some things I was missing, or some blockages I still needed to work on.

I struggled for many months, trying to work on these things, but life and work were busy, and it became kind of easy to put the "healing" aside.

Then, the craziest thing happened. I was invited to a friend's work party. I wouldn't have thought twice about going, but it was going to be in one of the trendiest/newest clubs in the city... no way would I get to experience that on my own, so I decided to go and have some fun.

And guess what? Yup. Call it fate, God, whatever... but I ended up meeting someone who I immediately knew was WAY out of my league. No way I would ever meet her in any other setting or situation. She didn't seem to notice that I could not keep up with her.

Over the next year, my entire life changed — in such amazing ways. It's hard to imagine I wasted so many years lost, alone, hurting — and not even knowing it.

I was introduced to additional healing, including changing my attitudes on food and exercise. And I still meditate and do breath-work exercises.

I feel like, after almost 50 years of being alive, I am FINALLY discovering who I am, why I am, and what I can still become. I sometimes get down, looking back at how many years I wasted being (if I am brutally honest) being really ignorant and unaware of just how much I did not know myself; or maybe being afraid to truly know myself. But those moments are fleeting because I really try to just stay in the present and just really have gratitude that I have now learned this much!

I am hurting again at the moment, because I lost my friend. I was not ready for that amazing love — and I now realize I was also not ready to give my love fully to another. But, I see so much hope, because I have finally learned that I am worthy of love and that I can give love — once I finally and fully love myself. *Not there yet.*

But I am excited! Another retreat has come into my purview... and I am about to put in my deposit for a true healing retreat in Costa Rica with a psychedelic spirit that I feel like is appearing in my dreams. So, in about six months, I will be having a long visit with Mother Ayahuasca in hopes of taking my healing to the purest and highest level.

I am already working on the Dieta I need to follow, according to the healing center. It doesn't have to start this early, but I have always had a major weakness for fried and sweet stuff... and I owe it to myself to clean up my eating and nutrition. I also hope to wean myself off social media and too much news...

This final leg of my healing journey, I hope, will set me up for the rest of my life, as long as I maintain it.

Final words:

If you feel something is off in your life, even if you don't remember anything bad happening to you, consider a healing journey. The self-discovery, in some ways, was more valuable to me than the healing — but I guess some would say the self-discovery was actually part of the healing.

Editor's Notes About Me'Shell's Healing Journey

- Trauma can be both something that happened to you OR something that was **withheld** from you. Because many people don't understand the second part of this definition, they don't think they experienced trauma in their lives. Truly, everyone can benefit from a healing journey.
- The most fascinating thing about healing and healing journeys is that the healing eventually finds you, perhaps finally at a time when you're ready. But you don't have to wait; you can be proactive in starting your healing journey.
- As pointed out throughout this book, there are a number of excellent healing modalities, though not all may work for you — or help with all the healing you need. Part of your healing journey is discovering what best works for you.
- It's never too late — nor too early — to begin a healing journey. The key is simply taking that first step and working at it, then working at it some more... and continuing that process, integrating all you learn, until you have joy, love, and peace in your life.

CHAPTER 30:
Healing Journey Story #11

Breathe More YOU

First Name: Marissa

Age: Xennial (Millennial/Gen X Cusp)

Gender: Female

How/Why You Started on Healing Journey: I began my healing journey after a series of life events (death, burnout, childbirth) had me questioning what I was doing with my life. I realized I had spent most of it trying to be "good" for others and didn't know what goodness meant for me. After an experience with my inner child, I began exploring how to nurture and protect myself instead of constantly abandoning myself for others.

Words That Describe Where You are in Your Healing Journey: Settling into the "messy middle," where I am not starting and definitely haven't finished. Every day is an inquiry of how to connect with myself and others so I am present, authentic, and loving. Currently, I am developing my capacity for acceptance and bringing it back to the basics with present moment awareness in the breath — taking that momentary pause to reflect in the moment. That breath can make the difference between an automatic response and the person you want to be.

Most Valuable Thing You've Learned on Your Healing Journey: Healing and self-care is an infinite journey; you'll never "arrive" until you've quite literally reached "the end" to take your last breath. Relating to it as one long roadtrip with twists and turns versus racing to a linear end can make it more enjoyable. T*ake* *rest breaks, enjoy the scenery, make sure you have enough gas, good tunes and companions you enjoy, and don't be afraid to re-direct when necessary.*

Progress on Your Healing Journey: I now relate to it as a practice. Initially, I think I thought if I did all the things and checked the boxes, I would be officially "healed" and would no longer feel certain things anymore. The human experience is a continually evolving spectrum and life will continue to throw punches. I continue to develop limits and boundaries relationally and with myself to take care of my nervous system. I've also been able to create flexibility with myself around play and doing less, breaking apart old stories of worthiness and "you can't have fun until the work is done" (which it never is!). I must admit my children are the best teachers for play!

Hardest Part of Your Healing Journey: Not everyone cares, gets it, or wants to heal. Hands down, this was the hardest part for me. It was devastating to have some of the most important people in my life tell me they didn't want to know about it, never mind try to understand it. To not have the opportunity to share myself felt like I was continuing with my façade of being a "good girl," and it was heartbreaking to know there was no desire on their end to actually "know me." When you choose to begin living authentically, in your full self, it can piss people off. Your behavior may no longer be convenient for them, or it brings up their own stuff and they react.

Best Advice to Someone Just Starting Their Healing Journey: Your healing is unique to you and will never look like anyone else's. It's so important to remember that your circumstances and season of life is different than others so comparing will bring tremendous suffering. Take what advice, tips and tricks can serve your present conditions and know you can always come back to the rest when things have evolved... it doesn't mean it's irrelevant, it's just not right now. Tiny habits consistently practiced over time, can lead to great change.

My Six Elements of Healing: What worked for me includes *psychedelics, breathwork, spirituality, nature, nutrition, and movement.*

My Healing Story:

"Well fancy meeting you here."

I would have stopped dead in my tracks to whirl around and see whose smug voice spoke that line, but I was breezing full tilt on my violet unicorn cruiser in a bike pack, on the Playa of Burning Man.

I nervously looked around as the voice was so audible it clearly had come from somewhere outside my head... but only, it hadn't. It definitely wasn't happening in reality, but the conversation was so vivid it may as well have been.

I pictured in my mind's eye, the owner of the voice as a little girl, no more than 7 years old eyeing me suspiciously with a smirk on her face. She sat on a swing, arms hanging on the ropes, toe in the dirt, twisting the swing side to side, her statement taunting me.

"Umm... well I can be here too." I timidly tried to work out the comment in my head, trying not to create attention from my bike-mates as I began a conversation with what appeared to be no one.

She snorted and rolled her eyes. *"Puh-leez!"*

"Well, I'm allowed to have fun too!" I noticed myself protesting and feeling attacked.

A big grin spread across her face *"You know, I could show you how to be happy if you'd just let me,"* she dared.

Straight to the gut, it felt like I was floating, time stood still. Every cell in my body knew it was true. I didn't even know how to have fun anymore.

I had just been marveling to myself about how beautiful this place, this moment was. Looking out at the horizon as we charged ahead on our bikes from one art installation to the other... The art, the music, Mother Nature, the freedom, and self-expression. The sheer awe of it felt like my heart was bursting, and then... I felt it.

Joy! A joy I had long since forgotten. I understood I was speaking to a younger version of myself. The part that knew how to play, create, and wonder. The part that knew grown-ups couldn't play their way out of a paper bag... and also knew, I was now an adult.

I felt my body soften and surrender. She was right, she did know, and I clearly didn't. I felt awkward and out of place.

All I could utter was a confused "What?"

"I could show you how to be happy, if you'd just let me." This time it came from inside me, an inner wisdom. It was kind, compassionate, and loving. It knew.

Trusting it, I agreed. "Okay then, I promise to let you show me. I promise to take care of you. We can go on play-dates and you can show me what makes you happy."

She smiled smugly, like she didn't quite believe me but also didn't care *"Deal."*

In that moment, with tears streaming down my face, I promised myself to take care of that little girl. I realized she had long been left behind in the rush to "grow up" and be responsible... and she was pissed with all the broken promises.

Sharing my first-time burn with others off the Playa, I was met with and incredulous "YOU went to Burning Man?!" and a "What drugs were you on?!" when sharing my moment of dialogue with this mysterious imagined little girl on a swing.

I found myself mildly irritated by people's reactions.

I mulled over what was nothing short of a transformational experience. Friends warned me I'd never be the same after, but I was shaken. I tried to pull apart the components of Burning Man that stacked together, made such a beautiful memorable experience. There was community, nature, art, movement, and, of course, psychedelics. (I did a lot of psychedelics that week, most for the first time ever in my life. I had always been a "if you can grow it, I'll do it" kind of gal but I took on a "When in Rome" motto for the week as I was dead set on experiencing of ALL Burning Man.)

Life back in the "default world" afterward was bumpy.

A Healing Journey Begins:

Nothing felt the same. I could no longer unsee what I had just seen and forget what I experienced on the Playa. What the hell happened? There were not many people I could talk about it with — I mean, I'm somebody's mother and a senior manager for a global beauty company, so it all seemed pretty risqué.

What was it about the Playa that made it so magical? What did little me want to do? How could I begin to bring these elements of Burning Man together in my everyday life?

My dates with little me started small and sadly. I had somehow neglected to take basic care of myself as an adult, so I began with journaling intentions and gratitude.

I took *little me* to yoga weekly. I discovered I didn't know how to be in my body. I didn't know how to move it, release it, or love it. Stuck all day in meetings and behind a desk, it would open and love me back with every twist, stretch, and savasana. I noticed myself being brought back each time to participate in community with my mat mates and favorite instructor.

Recalling the breathtaking heat from the Playa, I also began exploring hot yoga. Sweating buckets, opening, releasing tension, and trusting myself in poses that I would want to just give up on, reminded me of the physiological and psychological stamina of the Playa mid-day.

I began hitting the elliptical in the office gym at lunch and listening to DJ sets from Burning Man. Most of my life, the gym was for working out so I could avoid looking terrible naked. I began to realize that the midday cardio and positive emotions that came along with the music made me less of an asshole in meetings, at home, and to myself.

I started putting myself in creative spaces — museums, festivals, and communities — where people were actively engaged in the act of creation. I had a new appreciation for art, and I found tremendous therapeutic benefits from collaging and took on engaging with others to wonder and explore how they too, could look at life through design.

I was incredibly curious as to what went down during my psychedelic experience and found it challenging to not only articulate it, but to share. Not exactly a topic for water cooler office talk, never mind dinner tables, I found myself in internet rabbit holes. I came across an article on the similarities of floatation tanks and the psychedelic experience. I was hooked and began exploring the various tanks and chambers of Los Angeles looking to replicate the experience.

Exploring different ways to create altered states of consciousness, it was only a matter of time before I hit meditation. Sure, it was always there, but I was terrible at it and felt like my fashion and personality didn't quite fit in with the quiet, cloaked, stereotypes. My mind went a hundred miles an hour and I sat there judging in an incessant inquiry of "Am I doing this right?"

Practicing being in the present moment, observing sensations and thoughts, detaching, and witnessing, and cultivating positive qualities such as compassion and gratitude made a noticeable difference in my life in all areas.

Around this time, a girlfriend of mine invited me to join her in a Kundalini yoga class, which was unlike anything I had ever experienced. As we breathed our way to the 11th minute of the "Ego Eradicator" it was clear... I had no clue about the relationship between breath, body, and mind.

My spirit was wild after class and all I could think about was "Maybe if I knew how to breathe like that, I could have birthed my baby." My firstborn's labor was overdue, days long, complicated, and ended up in an emergency c-section. The more I explored the relationship between my mind and body, the more I could see how my fear added to the complications.

The felt experience of joy from Burning Man was my north star, and instead of scanning for risks, I found myself scanning for opportunities, to curate it for myself.

Exploring various modalities to mimic Playa experiences was an adventure and I found myself traipsing all over Los Angeles wishing there was something closer and more convenient... something that had it all. I wondered why wasn't there something that had these modalities under one roof.

I always thought if I ever left my company, it would be to open a studio, but my heart was never in it — until now. Instead of curating beauty on the outside, *I'd look to help others create it on the inside for themselves with a wellness studio.*

I moved my family home to Canada, to life a spend of life more in line with our values. We stayed with my folks on their farm in Manitoba while we shopped for a new Canadian city, and I studied meditation and worked on my business plan.

When the world shut down for the Covid-19 virus, I leaned hard into Mother Nature, creating community with our animals, grounding through gardening, and creating a ritual of moon walks.

One of the silver linings from the pandemic is it brought the world online seemingly overnight. Suddenly I had access to conferences and education I never would have been able to participate in given my location. I couldn't get enough of the world of psychedelics and the amazing research and studies that were coming out. It felt like this was what I intuitively knew but couldn't articulate to others.

Then I came across a podcast from one of my former LA meditation studios and they were interviewing a gentleman who teaches breathwork. I found the guy so relatable — he was sharp and quick-witted, and demystified the breath. Jon Paul Crimi developed his own unique style and quickly began selling out breathwork classes all over Los Angeles; one of the pioneers in breathwork.

Another pioneer is Wim Hof — and his phrase "get high on your own supply" had me take notice of breathwork and its similarity to psychedelics, but I've been unable to explore fully until now. Given big breathwork practices aren't recommended during pregnancy, I'd been waiting to explore it and now with online accessibility I could participate from my home in the middle of nowhere!

My first experience was wild! The physical, emotional, and mental release was unlike anything I had ever experienced.

I felt like I had the physical experience of having gone for a run and the emotional release of a big cry. For once my mind was quiet.... well at first it was pissed, but I was able to turn inward and connect to my breathing technique and the judgment was no longer there. I was able to visualize without the constant baratement and fully experience compassion, gratitude, and love again.

It was also the closest I had ever come to mimicking the psychedelic experience.

Still, I deeply yearned for the mystical experience that a psychedelic medicine ceremony provides and hoped to get some answers on what next steps could look like for me in this space of unclarity. One day, with my parents out of town for a doctor visit, I seized the opportunity to sit with psylocibin! I pulled together all the information I had learned from conferences, books, and podcasts on creating set and setting. My room was transformed into a beautiful ceremonial space, and just like with breathwork, I tuned out the outside world with my eye mask and a playlist borrowed from Johns Hopkins.

The visions were beautiful and vivid, and I had built enough trust with myself and my breath to surrender to the visions and their lessons. Every time I saw something that would alert fear in my body I'd anchor into my breath, low and slow, and use the word "surrender" as my mantra.

There wasn't an instruction manual in my visions to get out of the uncomfortable experience I was finding myself in these days, but rather I found myself loosening my grip on the outcome. An acceptance in something bigger, beyond my reality was at play, and was looking to create something magical if only I'd allow it.

Shortly after my sit with psilocybin, I decided to make the move from being owner/operator of a brick-and-mortar wellness studio, to a breathwork and meditation guide of an online one.

I felt like the world didn't need another online yoga teacher, but if I could help others metabolize the difficult emotions they were experiencing while stuck at home, I could contribute to healing. I was full of difficult emotions, and I was slowly learning they were becoming my best teachers — grief and rage specifically. Much like ghosts, these emotions wanted just to be witnessed and acknowledged before moving on.

My previous coping strategy of numbing out with wine and weed; definitely not the person who was cracked open on the playa by JOY.

One particularly memorable breathwork session, I was filled with a rage and fury I immediately knew wasn't mine. Recalling my psychedelic experience, I turned toward it and surrendered to the breath letting it carry us along. This thundering rage seemed to be from the women who came before me, those who were misunderstood and lost their voices in the systems of patriarchal oppression. Those who looked to the sun, moon and stars, who looked to the land for healing and inward for trust in their sense of self and intuition... those who were eventually burned at the stake.

It was the catalyst that had me begin exploring spirituality newly, far from the dogmatic approach I had been raised with. The ability to turn inward and witness the divine in myself, others, and all around was something no organized religion had ever been able to teach.

As I continue to shed old ways of being and create new ones, it becomes increasingly challenging to abandon myself in the interest of living up to the expectations of others. I'm continually learning to honor people where they're at and respect where folks are on their spiritual journey knowing it's not for the faint of heart.

Recently I was met with some more of life's "speed-bump-learning-curves" and took the opportunity to join a group psilocybin experience. I had gone into ceremony seeking how I could be of service to the world and found myself on a play date with my inner child — this time she trusted me. She took me deeper into visions and places I might not have fully understood or been willing to accept that day on the playa in 2017.

Through healing, I've learned to respect my spiritual journey and how to trust, using the breath to surrender to all of it. The key take-away from my ceremony: **"Be more YOU."**

Editor's Notes About Marissa's Healing Journey

- It's extremely valuable to consider using ALL of the healing modalities. They often work well together, but also have individual strengths. Keep experimenting.
- No comparisons! Don't compare your trauma nor your healing journey to anyone else's. Everyone has their own experiences. Make YOUR healing YOUR focus.
- Almost all healing journeys involve some time healing our inner child — and rediscovering that childlike joy and wonder... and PLAY.
- Breathwork is a practice that can be developed into an extremely mind-expanding and consciousness-growing experience.
- Wim Hof found he could enhance his performance through developing a command his body, breath, and mind using specific breathing techniques and tolerance to extreme temperatures. His breathing work has been shown to help with depression, anxiety, mood, mental focus, and pain management.

Marissa Kosolofski is a psychedelic advocate, community builder, and the creatrix of The Golden Thread Studio, an online wellness studio specializing in breathwork journeys and self-care practices. Learn more at her website: www.thegoldenthreadstudio.com.

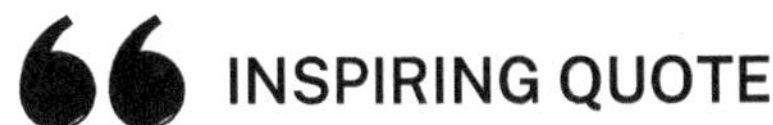

"What happens when people open their hearts? They get better." —Haruki Murakami

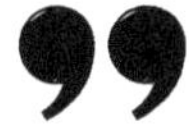

PART FOUR:

HEALING QUICK SHEETS

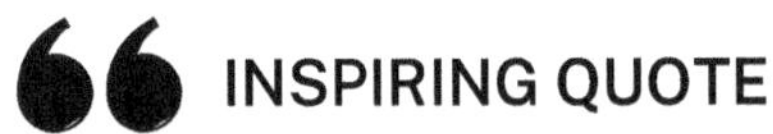

"Each of us has a unique part to play in the healing of the world." —Marianne Williamson

CHAPTER 31:
Five Keys to Healing; Finding Your True Whole Self

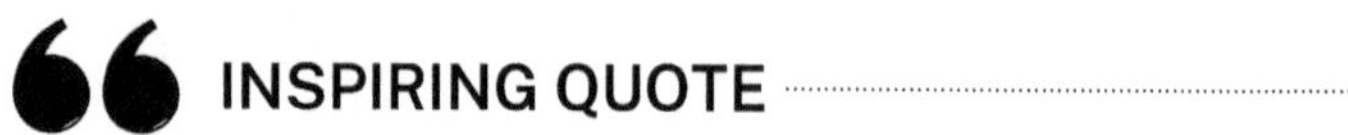

INSPIRING QUOTE

"The privilege of a lifetime is to become who you truly are." — Carl Jung

It's time, right? Time to find your true path — the path to your authentic self.

But finding the true you and your true purpose takes healing — authentic and complete healing, not a Band-Aid of self-medicating and/or prescription medicines.

There's no time like the present to complete your research on healing and to start making moves to begin the journey of discovering (or rediscovering) your true self... your WHOLE self.

GOAL: START A HEALING JOURNEY WITH THE GOAL OF CLEARING TRAUMA, RAISING CONSCIOUSNESS, AND BECOMING WHOLE.

1. **Patience: The Healing Journey Takes Time.** There are no speed limits along your healing journey, but know that for most people, it takes time. The more trauma you have to process, the longer your healing journey. The key is patience and understanding that healing is a process that sets its own pace. And as one colleague states, "In reality, your healing journey is never really over until you're dead."

2. **Determination: The Healing Journey Takes Work.** Make no mistake, a healing journey is hard work. Think of healing like peeling the layers of an onion: each layer must be healed before moving to the next layer of unhealed trauma responses. Believe me, the hard work is amazingly worth it — because leading an authentic and true life is worth it. There's no magic pill or wand for healing — except the magic inside you that will help sustain your healing journey.

3. **Tenderness: The Healing Journey Takes Love.** We tend to be our own harshest critics, which is partly why some of us are here now — because we're the ones bullying ourselves! A healing journey is NOT linear, so expect progress as well as setbacks... but with those setbacks, be gentle on yourself and show yourself love and compassion. It's also important to have community to support and love on you as you make this critical journey.

4. **Healing Tools: The Healing Journey Takes Multiple Modalities.** One of the most important lessons about healing journeys is that most of us will need to use (and continue to use) more than one healing modality. Furthermore, all these healing modalities are related and work well together. But it's also important to remember that healing is multidimensional. For example, you can't heal your mind while eating garbage food or being sedentary.

5. **Integration: The Healing Journey Must be Fully Assimilated.** The most important part of the healing journey, as you start the healing, is creating a system to help you integrate all the things you discover about your true self. By healing, you may need to make minor or major changes in your life regarding the people, lifestyle, and work. Integration is often a combination of individual work (often through something like journaling) and reflective work with your people and/or a coach or therapist.

CHAPTER 32:

Five Healthy Ways to Practice Self-Care

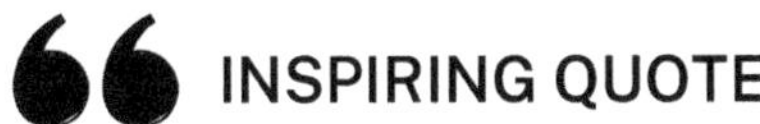

"When we care for ourselves as our very own beloved — with naps, healthy food, clean sheets, a lovely cup of tea — we can begin to give in wildly generous ways to the world, from abundance." — Anne Lamott

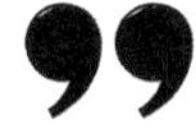

Often when we are deep in our trauma, deep in the hurt and depression, we tend to forget about taking care of ourselves — and that's what self-care is about. It's not about being selfish or over-indulgent; self-care is about supporting yourself, putting up healthy boundaries, and providing a space for healing.

Self-care is about nourishing yourself... nourishing your body, emotions, mind, and spirit. Self-care isn't a tool for healing, but it is a tool for helping you cope when the trauma or healing from the trauma weighs you down. Self-care is a great tool for giving us a short-term boost to keep moving through our healing journey.

Experts suggest that a regular self-care routine may help build self-esteem and confidence, reduce generalized anxiety and stress, and improve overall happiness. In the long-term, self-care can help foster healing, manage chronic illness, improve interpersonal relationships, and may play a role in the prevention of future diseases (according to a 2017 study from the American Heart Association).

GOAL: BEGIN INCORPORATING A SELF-CARE ROUTINE TO YOUR DAILY LIFE.

1. **Daily Self-Care.** Find moments throughout the day to focus on things/people to be grateful for; take short walks in nature; snuggle with a pet or loved one; enjoy a special treat; set boundaries with people; step outside and watch the stars; use a weighted blanket; shut off your social media; cook yourself a delicious meal; chat with a friend or loved one; listen/sing/dance to your favorite music.

2. **Emotional Self-Care.** Tap into tools to keep your emotions operating at an even keel. Use affirmations or other positive self-talk and encouragement; schedule fun times with friends; plan a vacation or getaway; take a break from the news and/or social media; keep a gratitude journal; talk with a coach or therapist; forgive someone who wronged you; nourish your inner child.

3. **Physical Self-Care.** Because our bodies play such a key role in healing and health, we also need to practice physical self-care. The focus here are techniques such as taking a nap when you're exhausted; obtaining better and regular sleep; focusing on eating healthy and nutritious foods; keeping to a weekly schedule of physical activity; enjoying a massage; taking a bath; dancing to your favorite songs; yoga.

4. **Spiritual Self-Care.** These things are fundamentally about connecting with and strengthening your inner spirit. They include attending religious services; praying; practicing forgiveness; meditating; joining a prayer group; spending time in nature/forest bathing; doing yoga; celebrating the seasons; volunteering for a cause you love.

5. **Mental Self-Care.** It's also important to nourish and love our brains, to help better manage our thoughts, and to keep negative self-talk at bay. Some examples include: reading a book; listening to a podcast; working at a hobby; learning a new language; visiting a museum; doing a puzzle; solving mind games/puzzles; creative writing and journaling; clearing clutter/organizing your living space.

CHAPTER 33:
Five Methods to Foster Self-Love

 **INSPIRING QUOTE**

"Believing in our hearts that who we are is enough is the key to a more satisfying and balanced life." — Ellen Sue Stern

It may sound obvious, but we have to truly value ourselves and love ourselves, before we can ever love anyone else or allow them to love us.

What is self-love? Think of it as self-respect, self-acceptance. It's not about having a huge ego or being a narcissist. It encompasses not only how we treat ourselves but also our thoughts and feelings about our self-worth.

When you love yourself — when you have self-love — you have an overall positive view of yourself. (This statement does not mean you feel great about yourself all the time; it simply means you feel your life is headed in the right direction, even with a few bumps in the road.) It's about embracing your full self, including your strengths and weaknesses, triumphs and challenges, successes and mistakes.

Self-love is essential in protecting ourselves from predators and others who seek to take advantage of people who don't value themselves. Also, without self-love, you may be self-sabotaging yourself.

When we have self-love, we are stronger, happier, and enjoy healthy, positive relationships.

GOAL: BUILD, ENHANCE ACCEPTANCE AND SELF-LOVE.

1. **Self-Acceptance is Crucial.** The first step in cultivating self-love is self-kindness and forgiving yourself of anything negative from the past. No one is perfect; we all make mistakes. We are on a path toward healing — and that's all that matters.

2. **Your Reality Does Not Need to be Perfect.** Your life might be a mess right now, you might be between romantic relationships or even not living in your ideal circumstances... but as long as you are safe and making progress on yourself, improving yourself, the surroundings shouldn't be a concern.

3. **Challenge and Dismiss Negative Thoughts.** Regardless of where we are on our healing journey, negative thoughts can pop up at any time; our goal should be to shut them down before they gain any momentum. Consider trying Loving-Kindness Meditation, which utilizes mantras that emphasize kindness toward oneself and others.

4. **Stop Comparing Yourself to Others.** The Comparison Syndrome is a real thing, and occurs when we compare our abilities, talents, and skills to others — and find ourselves lacking. It's especially bad when we compare ourselves to unrealistic air-brushed images of models, but it can happen simply as we scroll through social media.

5. **Establish Clear Boundaries in Relationships.** When you don't have self-love, people will run you over, take advantage of you, and treat you like nothing. Many of us have a difficult time saying no because we don't have boundaries. You need to establish rules to protect yourself... to protect your physical, emotional, energy, time, and financial resources.

CHAPTER 34:

Five Natural Tools for Better Sleep

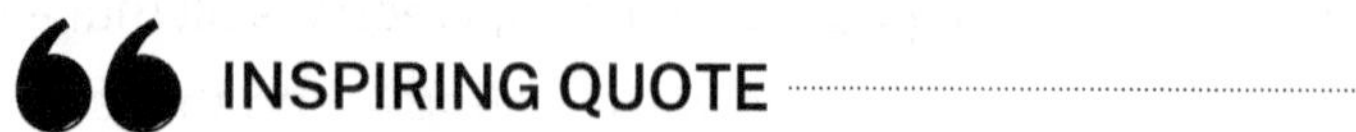

INSPIRING QUOTE

"A good laugh and a long sleep are the best cures in the doctor's book." —Irish proverb

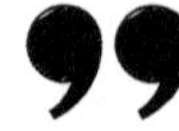

Sleep is essential to good health... and your path toward healing.

That said, about a third of us — perhaps more — suffer from insomnia. Those of us suffering from depression, anxiety, and PTSD are even more likely to suffer with insomnia.

Please do not be the 10 percent or so that go the conventional route and obtain a prescription for a sleep aid. It doesn't matter which; all these drugs are absolutely horrible... and the over-the-counter types are just as bad.

Why take chemical compounds with sometimes dangerous side effects just to get sleep? Because we know how important sleep is to our health — but the pills and liquids should be avoided at all costs.

GOAL: OBTAIN BETTER SLEEP WITH ONE OR MORE NATURAL SLEEP AIDS.

1. **Cannabis.** Hands down, this plant works miracles with sleep and pain. If you live in a state with medical or recreational cannabis sales, then seek out a tincture (or edible) created for sleep. You can also look into one or more CBD products legally produced from hemp. Many producers make blends specifically for sleep, pain relief, recovery.

2. **GABA.** One of the trendier natural sleep aids is Gamma-aminobutyric acid (GABA), an amino acid that reduces the activity in brain cells. GABA is a neurotransmitter that inhibits brain activity, helping with sleep. Some small trials have shown that supplementing with GABA can reduce stress and relax the mind, thus allowing people to fall asleep more easily.

3. **Valerian Root.** A perennial flowering grassland plant native to Europe and Asia seems to reduce the amount of time it takes to fall asleep AND sleep better. Valerian has been used for centuries as a medicine for numerous ailments. People have used valerian root to treat migraines, tiredness, stomach cramps, and insomnia.

4. **Kava.** Also known as kava kava, here's another herb that is mainly used for reducing anxiety, but also as a sleep aid because of its calming effects on the mind and body. Kava is rich in kavalactones, chemicals that can have a sedative (sleep-inducing) effect by reducing stress and anxiety.

5. **California Poppy.** These beautiful flowers, cousins of the more infamous poppies, grow all over the Pacific Northwest (and elsewhere). This plant seems to be the newest medicinal plant, touted for its anti-anxiety, mild pain relief, and sleep-inducing effects — though it has been known in folk medicine circles for its sedative properties.

Other non-prescription options you might also want to consider: chamomile, passionflower, St. John's Wort, magnesium, magnolia bark, Vitamin D, and 5-HTP.

Note: *The hormone melatonin was left off this list because there are many mixed feelings about it and its side effects. Read more here: https://healthresearchfunding.org/pros-cons-melatonin/*

CHAPTER 35:
Five Easy Ways to Cultivate Gratitude

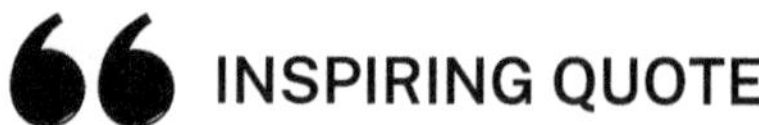

INSPIRING QUOTE

"While your brain is wired to seek out the negative to keep you safe, gratitude is a simple way to rewire your brain to see the bigger picture." — Ashleigh Edelstein, LMFT

Even in the most trying situations, we can usually convince ourselves to find something we can appreciate — something for which we can express gratitude; thus, gratitude is an emotion similar to appreciation and thankfulness. The word comes from the Latin *gratus*, which means "pleasing" or "thankful."

Instead of turning to unhealthy coping mechanisms when you are feeling badly — such as self-medicating, binge drinking, chowing down on junk food, compulsive shopping — instead turn to something that can be permanently rewarding: practicing gratitude.

Often times when we are hurting, what we need most is a change — and gratitude changes your perspective of yourself and your place in the world.

Remember that line many of us hear as children? "Count your many blessings" — that's gratitude.

Gratitude helps improve our self-esteem, sleep patterns, and physical and mental health... and expressing gratitude to others helps spread the love and joy to others.

GOAL: SET AN INTENTION TO BE MORE MINDFUL OF THINGS AND PEOPLE TO BE GRATEFUL FOR IN YOUR LIFE.

1. **Keep a Gratitude Journal.** Set a daily practice of writing (or recording) the positive elements of your life — helping remind yourself of the gifts, people, and good things you enjoy. If you have ever journaled previously, the key here is making it a habit — a daily habit. It's amazing how focusing on the positive moves you toward healing.

2. **Gratitude Prompts.** Before some of us can even start thinking on our own about gratitude, we may need to supplement our practice with prompts to help us focus on gratitude. Considers prompts such as:

   - Five things I like about myself
   - The most beautiful part of my day
   - Three things I am thankful for today
   - People in my life who bring me joy

3. **Mindfulness/Living in the Present.** The daily grind of life can be challenging and exhausting... even overbearing. A really great tool to develop is building mindfulness moments into your daily schedule, ideally once every hour, but you don't need to be so rigid; the key is taking a few minutes, several times daily, of finding little things for which you are grateful.

4. **Meditation/Prayer.** In just about all spiritual and religious traditions, there are prayers and petitions of gratitude and thanksgiving. There are numerous guided meditations for gratitude as well — to appreciate what makes us feel good. We know the power of prayer and meditation for healing — they evoke a relaxation response that quells stress and quiets the body — allowing for gratitude to emerge.

5. **Gratitude Collage.** I love the idea of having a board where you can post pictures of all the things and people that are a positive force in your life. Not only is creating the collage a tool of gratitude, but the collage also becomes a visual reminder that can trigger thoughts of gratitude.

CHAPTER 36:
Five Strategies to Let Go of Control and Surrender

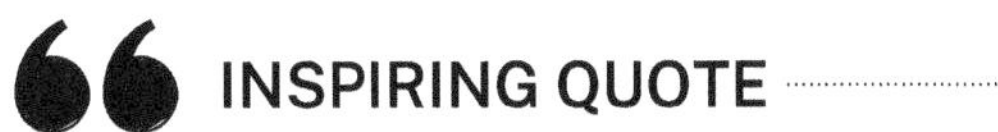

INSPIRING QUOTE

"Surrender is a journey from outer turmoil to inner peace." — Sri Chinmoy

Surrender is the goal; it's a win, not a weakness. It's the moment when you decide to stop the in-fighting that is going on within you because of the trauma you have experienced.

Our egos are often a bit out of control — even (or more especially because) when we have experienced trauma and are deep in it. Our ego feels a need to protect us and will go into overdrive to do so; our ego can be the proverbial brick wall we hit when dealing with unprocessed trauma. (That said, our ego is also the thing that protects us, so it is a fine balance here.)

If we are to heal, though, we need to push that ego aside and surrender to those unprocessed emotions (our fears and negative patterns) so that we can release them — the key to the healing process.

The problem is that the ego does not really want to relinquish control, and will hold on for as long as possible — until the point of pure pain and exhaustion.

Surrendering is about accepting that you will need to make a change of perspective in your worldview. Surrendering is about totally letting go and allowing emotions, thoughts, and actions to simply flow, often without direction at first. Surrendering takes practice, so be patient with yourself.

Finally, when we truly surrender, the result that follows often includes feelings of relief, gratitude, grace, and sometimes even joy.

GOAL: FIND THE KEY TOOLS THAT HELP YOU SURRENDER TO HEALING.

1. **Make a Paradigm Shift.** At some point, you simply must make a radical change in your thinking. Do the research, talk with experts, and forge a path to a new way of thinking that allows you to surrender those old ways of thinking.

2. **Work With a Coach or Therapist.** Many of us need a helping hand to quiet the ego, and a healing coach or therapist might be the key to finding a way of letting go and surrendering. Having an ally in your corner might be just what you need to find the strength to surrender.

3. **Pray or Meditate.** To me, the greatest peace I have ever felt — and continue to feel — is when I surrendered all my "stuff" to God. It's when we pass all our troubles, anxiety, control to the Divine, it provides such a release. We can do this as a prayer or a meditation.

4. **Take a Psychedelic Journey.** A heavy dose of intentional psychedelic medicine is often enough to push your ego aside so you can move right into healing mode, BUT, even with these powerful medicines, people still need to acknowledge surrendering to it.

5. **Embrace It.** Start with something like "I choose to surrender to..." or "If I completely surrender, what would my life look like." Create a mindset or intention that you will begin this healing journey by slowly implementing this plan.

CHAPTER 37:
Five Methods to Get in More Daily/ Weekly Exercise

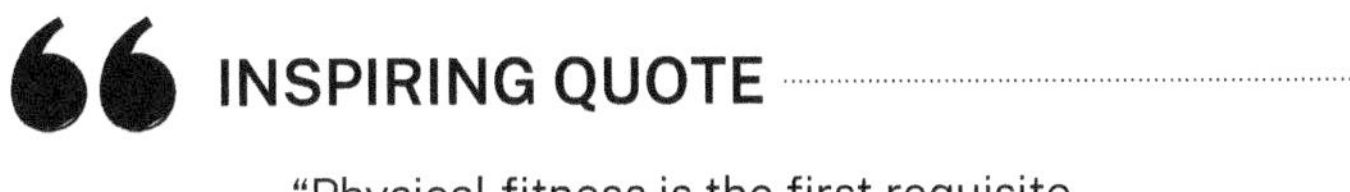

INSPIRING QUOTE

"Physical fitness is the first requisite of happiness." — Joseph Pilates

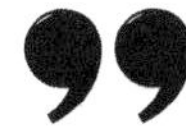

We often overthink elements of life — and exercise is one of them. You don't need expensive equipment or a gym membership; you simply need the mindset.

GOAL: SET AN INTENTION OF DOING SOME AMOUNT OF EXERCISE DAILY; THE BENEFITS ARE ENORMOUS.

1. **Just Do It!** Yes, the Nike slogan rings true. Set a daily routine to walk, bike, swim, stretch, workout. Find something you like doing — and do it every day. For many years, when I had dogs, I would walk them a minimum of 2 miles each morning; not only was it great exercise in nature, but I found I had to take my phone with me to record "brilliant" ideas that the walking and silence brought forth.
2. **Make it Part of Your Workday.** Whether you are working from home or back in the office, make exercise breaks part of your daily routine. If working from home, take breaks to vacuum, garden, clean. If commuting to work, maybe you walk or bike to the train station — or simply a few laps around your block, if working from home. My partner Jenny used to take two daily 15 minute breaks that involved walking the nature paths right outside her workplace.

3. **Park Far Away From the Store.** Or, better, consider walking or riding your bike to the store. Every time I need to shop at a local big box store, I am constantly amazed how many people cut through the parking lots to try and find the one close spot, even circling several times. I park at the far end of the lot, where almost no one parks, and enjoy a nice stroll to the store.

4. **Use the Stairs.** Walking is perhaps the best overall exercise, but I think close behind is walking up and down the stairs — of your workplace, your home or apartment. You don't need a stair machine; and if you don't have stairs anywhere, you might consider using a small (and sturdy) crate or buying a few step platforms.

5. **Have a Dance Party.** One of the best forms of exercise is dance — and who doesn't love to get into the groove of a good song? So, take a break from your screen, crank up the volume, and dance up a storm — even better if you can enlist a partner or coworker to join in! And, of course, you could also sign up for dancing, utilizing businesses that offer Jazzercise or Zumba or others.

Bottomline: Find the things that you like doing — and do them regularly. Besides the cardio (of which you can stay light to moderate or go deep with your doctor's approval), you should also add a strength component to your weekly routine. Finally, combine exercise/moving your body with something else you enjoy; for me, that includes working in the forest, trail clearing, litter pickup... physical activity in nature.

CHAPTER 38:

Five Suggestions for Developing/ Finding Community

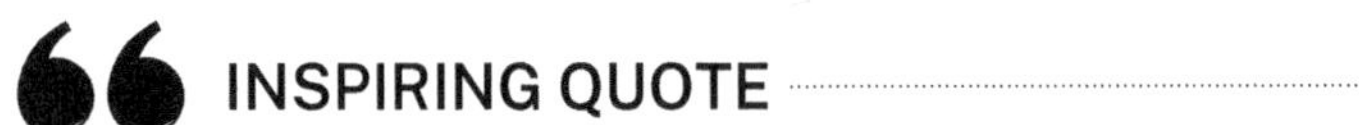

INSPIRING QUOTE

"The need for connection and community is primal, as fundamental as the need for air, water, and food." —Dean Ornish

We are not a solitary species. We are meant to interact with others, to love and laugh and share with people who mean something to us. In doing so, we actually improve our health—and with support of our community (our tribe, our people), we have more strength and resilience.

Community anchors us, provides meaning, and results in joy. What is community? The simplest answer is that community is a group of people, but it's what binds the people together in community that is key.

Finding, building, joining community takes work—often, a lot of time and effort.

Here's the key: When you start to make dramatic changes to your life, when you find true healing, you NEED to have a community supporting you, supporting your healing, supporting your new life.

GOAL: SET AN INTENTION OF FINDING YOUR PEOPLE.

1. **Start Local.** Generally speaking, there are many groups right in your community. There are probably any number of clubs (for sports, cards, crafts, etc.), events (book clubs, sporting events, speakers), and religious/worship groups that are always looking for new members. Ask around, visit your local library, or find your community newspaper/website for more ideas and information.

2. **Meetup.** One of the best ways to find groups of like-minded people — either locally or across the globe — is Meetup. Founded about 20 years ago, Meetup is a social media platform for hosting and organizing in-person and virtual activities, gatherings, and events for people and communities of similar interests, hobbies, and professions. It's free for users, and there are literally thousands of groups to choose from — both local and remote.

3. **Online Communities.** Depending on your needs and interests, there are numerous online communities in which you might find community. Go to your favorite search engine, which should be Ecosia (because they protect your privacy AND plant trees for every search), and search for groups. You can also gain some insights by reading this article from Psychedelic Passage: "How to Find a Psychedelic Community Near Me." (https://www.psychedelicpassage.com/how-to-find-a-psychedelic-community-group-near-me/)

4. **Social Media Groups.** Both Facebook and LinkedIn have groups you can join based on your interests and profession. There are company-focused groups, sales groups, and issue-themed groups. Make sure you read the group's description

and rules before joining. Most groups allow an introduction, so plan it out and take it slowly.

5. **Volunteering.** The true win-win of community is volunteering. Nonprofit organizations are almost always in need of volunteers and by joining one that aligns with your values and interests, you will find like-minded folks who are giving back to the community. For example, I volunteer with a group that supports my local library and also with a local land conversancy organization focused on protecting the health of a key watershed.

CHAPTER 39:
Five Approaches to Foster Forgiveness

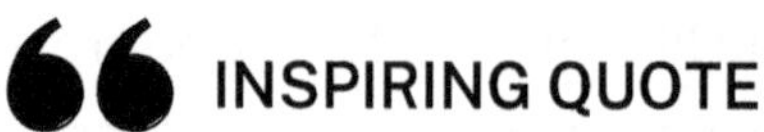

INSPIRING QUOTE

"The weak can never forgive. Forgiveness is the attribute of the strong." —Mahatma Gandhi

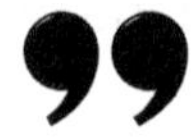

Forgiveness is one of those tough ones, right? We've been hurt, abused, and wounded — so why should we be the one offering forgiveness? But that's the wrong perspective. The pain of living with unforgiveness can poison your soul and destroy you, so it really becomes your only choice.

When we talk about forgiveness, it's two-pronged. Yes, you are truly forgiving the person who hurt you, but the psychological benefits for US in forgiveness are immense; forgiving helps give us a new sense of strength and self-esteem, as well as decreasing depression, resentment, anxiety, anger, and PTSD.

Forgiveness is important for our overall health. Forgiveness helps reduce our stress levels, improve our immune system, heart-health, sleep, and self-esteem.

Forgiveness is not about letting someone off the hook for their actions; it simply means choosing to let go of your anger, hurt, and desire for vengeance. Forgiveness is about finding peace.

Working on forgiveness can help lessen the grip of the memory on you; it can help free you from the control of the person who harmed you. Forgiveness is NOT about forgetting the trauma or excusing the abuser; nor do you have to face or forgive the person directly.

As a Christian, God commands that we forgive others and extend the grace that we have been shown in the forgiveness of our sins.

GOAL: FORGIVE THOSE WHO HURT US, INCLUDING OURSELVES.

1. **Forgive For Yourself.** Forgiveness is a gift you are giving to yourself; in fact, the person you're forgiving does not even need to know you have forgiven them. Forgiveness is not weak, it's freeing.

2. **Name It, Don't Blame It.** The blame-game is a fun one; we can spend hours going down the blame rabbit hole, when our goal with forgiveness should be to identify it — and release its hold on us.

3. **Take Action to Move On.** Reframe everything. Move your thinking from victim to survivor; from helpless to empowered. You are strong, you are healing, you are not your trauma.

4. **Practice Mindfulness/Gratitude.** Changing your focus/perspective from the negative to the positive in your life can help you move forward with forgiveness. We all have things to be grateful for — and it's good practice to focus on the positive.

5. **Compassion & Kindness.** Nobody is perfect, and while we like being on our righteous pedestal, it's healthier for us to focus on being compassionate — and forgiving. So many abusers were abused themselves; we know intergenerational abuse and trauma run strong.

Finally, if you are still struggling with forgiveness after reading this book, still deep in your trauma, consider joining a support group or seeing a therapist.

CHAPTER 40:
Five Paths to Finding/ Bringing More Joy

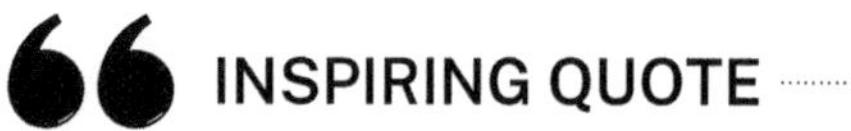

"I cannot even imagine where I would be today were it not for that handful of friends who have given me a heart full of joy. Let's face it, friends make life a lot more fun." — Charles R. Swindoll

We can have more joy in life, even if we are just starting on our healing journey, if we allow it. Sometimes with unprocessed trauma, it is hard to find joy or happiness.

What is joy? How is it different from happiness? Joy is a lasting internal reaction, a sense of peace, pleasure, and contentment about who you are, what you do, and the loving people in your life. Joy is lasting. Happiness is typically temporary and is often triggered by external events, people, and things.

GOAL: SET AN INTENTION OF FOCUSING ON BRINGING MORE JOY INTO YOUR LIFE.

1. **Heal and Let Go of the Past.** You'll have much greater joy once you are further along your healing journey and can put that trauma into the past. Our past does not define us nor does our age, gender, race, etc., limit us accomplishing what we love. The key here, as you are healing, is to identify the things, work, and people that bring you joy — and focus on those.

2. **Create Positive Daily Rituals.** I work from home and when I am writing, I could sit in my chair all day long, but that's not good for me — so I take 5 minute breaks, typically every hour. But it's not just a stretch break; I use the time to walk to a window and take a long gratitude moment. In the spring, I open a window to hear the Robin's song. The key is to find your positivity rituals. A friend of mine keeps a gratitude journal, while another attempts a daily act of kindness to both friends and strangers.

3. **Follow a Healing Protocol.** You will not have reliable joy in your life if you do not have self-love and are not healing. So, you should be looking at what you're eating, how much you're exercising, how much nature and sunlight you're getting, and how much spirituality/meditation/prayer you're doing. In other words, you need to be following the protocols listed earlier in the book.

4. **Cull/Cultivate Healthy Relationships (Including With Your Social Media Usage).** Why do we so often allow negative people to have so much influence/power over our lives? Why is so much of social media either fake happiness or pure hate — or so it seems. To be joyful, you need loving, supportive people in your life.

5. **Give Back/Pay It Forward.** In my mind, nothing gives me more joy than helping someone else, making their life better or easier. We can do this by simply offering our time and attention; and if you have the financial resources, donating money in addition to your time. The easiest way to do this is with your friends and family, but there are lots of articles with ideas for "paying it forward." By the way, adopting and caring for a pet, making their life better, fits as well.

CHAPTER 41:
Five Ways to Integrate Your Healing Journey

INSPIRING QUOTE

"Health is a state of complete harmony of the body, mind, and spirit. When one is free from physical disabilities and mental distractions, the gates of the soul open." — B.K.S. Iyengar

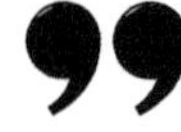

Let's start with a big round of applause for walking (crawling?) through your healing journey. It takes bravery to face the shadows and pains of your past to clear the road for a healthy future.

Congratulations on making the journey.

But your healing journey is not over; it never truly is. The next step is maintaining that healing, weaving your healing into ALL aspects of your life.

That weaving experience is what we call **integration**, which comes from the Latin word *integrare*, which means to form or blend into a whole, or to complete.

As you near the end of your healing journey, the work continues because you basically have two lives you need to merge/separate — the trauma-fueled life you led prior to healing and this new and beautiful life that is just starting.

The integration period is a tender time for people. We have gained insight into healing and have hopefully cleared most of our trauma, but now we need to relearn how to deal with LIFE!

GOAL: FOSTER AN INTENTION TO FULLY INTEGRATE YOUR HEALING JOURNEY INTO YOUR NEW LIFE.

1. **Find Your Community, Your Tribe, Your People.** As you begin your healing journey — and certainly by the time you are ready to start integrating it — you should examine your circle of friends, especially that inner circle. You'll most likely want to cultivate new people that will help support your healing journey, while ending things with others that are not helping your healing journey. Having a supportive community is essential to healing.

2. **Keep a Journal.** Make it a video, audio, or print journal, but just do it. Journaling is simply the easiest and best way to get your words out there. Write about the changes, the insights, the good, the bad, the setbacks, the triumphs... all these things are part of your healing journey. A few journaling prompts:

    - What attitudes and behaviors are no longer serving me?
    - What am I holding onto — and what can I let go?
    - What changes (including people, places, work) might I have to make in my new life?
    - Does my current work align with my newly discovered self? If not, what kind of work will fit?

3. **Try Meditating.** You already know meditation as a key spiritual healing modality, but it's also a great tool for integrating your healing. For example, there is a *Loving-Kindness Meditation*, which uses mantras that emphasize kindness toward ourself and others. (Learn more here: https://positivepsychology.com/loving-kindness-meditation/)

4. **Be Creative.** Some people dance, some draw or paint, but the idea is to express your healing journey through some creative outlet that provides you with positive reinforcement and joy.
5. **Consider a Coach or Therapist.** You may already be working with a coach or therapist, but if not, and you're struggling a bit with integrating your healing journey, then find an expert who can help you achieve your goals.

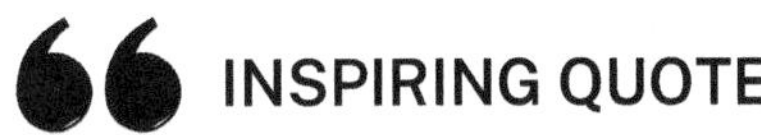

"Of one thing I am certain, the body is not the measure of healing, peace is the measure." — Phyllis McGinley

PART FIVE:
CONCLUSIONS AND HEALING RESOURCES

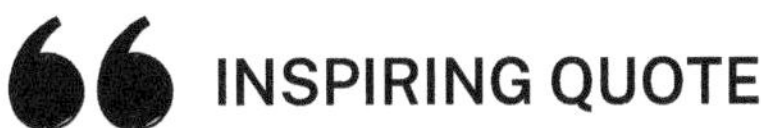

"Love one another and help others to rise to the higher levels, simply by pouring out love. Love is infectious and the greatest healing energy." — Sai Baba

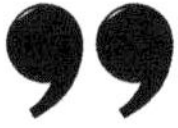

CHAPTER 42:
Conclusions on Healing... and Finding Your TRUE You

My hope is that you have been empowered and inspired by the content in this book to begin your own healing journey. I understand it can be daunting, scary, time-consuming, even risky — but if you want to live your true, authentic — and WHOLE — life, you need to start walking that journey.

We know our trauma is making us SICK. When we have unprocessed emotions stemming from trauma trapped within us, we tend toward extremely selfish and oftentimes self-destructive and pleasure-seeking behaviors and lifestyles. It also creates a wall around our hearts that prevents us from truly loving ourselves — or others.

People with trauma:

- Have issues with food (either overeating or undereating; almost always poor eating)
- Have issues with exercise (either immobilized or pushing to the extreme)
- Have issues with relationships (either isolating or with improper relationships)
- Have issues with self-love (typically self-loathing, but sometimes pleasure-seeking)
- Have issues regulating emotions (surfacing as angry outbursts, shame, fear, guilt)
- Have issues with health/illness (depression, anxiety, addiction, OCD, PTSD)

BUT, our trauma does not need to define us; our trauma is not our lot in life. Our trauma can be overcome... with intention, work, and integration.

We MUST take our healing into our own hands, minds, hearts, and spirits. We cannot rely on the conventional medical system — which focuses more on reducing symptoms than curing — to heal us or the people we love.

HEALING HINT

We MUST break the cycle that "pleasure traps" hold on us. The first part is healing your trauma. The second part is realizing what you should be seeking is joy, which comes from within us, and not happiness, which is a fleeting emotion. We need to eliminate these unnecessary "highs" from foods, drugs, sex, etc., that we erroneously think is our reward for living.

But we can't rely on the conventional food system either, as food labeling laws are vague, allowing marketers to make wild claims about products being "natural" that are actually full of toxic chemicals. Worse, we have marketers who are using and manipulating questionable ingredients to get us hooked on their low-quality, nutrient-weak foods. By consuming these hyperpalatable "food" products, we are unwittingly sabotaging our own health!

Many of us have had a vague sense of many of these health issues, but have continued to live an unhealthy lifestyle — too much reliance on the medical community for treatments, too much unhealthy eating, too little exercise/movement, or too little time spent in nature... on top of an unhealthy work-life balance and screen-life balance.

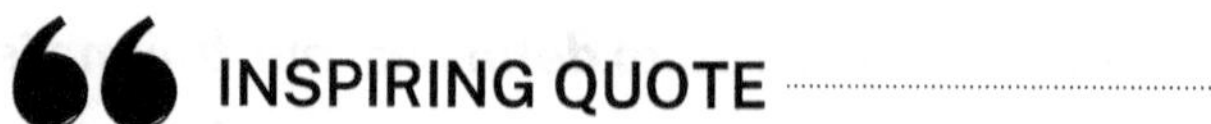

INSPIRING QUOTE

"The body heals with play, the mind heals with laughter, and the spirit heals with joy." —Proverb

That said, you must WANT healing. There's nothing that can be done for someone who wants to stay in the realm of suffering, who won't take actions to help themselves. Healing takes work; there is no magic pill that will cure us.

We live in a world that is:

- Overstimulated (bombarded)
- Fake (advertising, social media)
- Polluted (air, water, soil)
- Saturated with chemicals (food, air, water, soil)
- Screen-heavy (phones, tablets, monitors, televisions)
- Focused on the wrong things
- Secular and fragmented
- Hazardous to our health and healing
- Making us SICK!

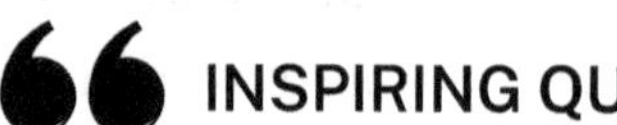

INSPIRING QUOTE

"Aboriginal healing practices are repetitive, rhythmic, relevant, relational, respectful, and rewarding — experiences known to be effective in altering neural systems involved in the stress response." — Bruce D. Perry, MD, PhD

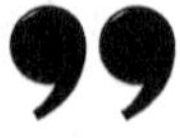

Are you ready to completely change your life for the BETTER? Are you ready to finally make the changes you need to heal, to remove all those masks we wear, to find (discover!) your authentic self? Are you ready to truly love yourself for the first time — and allow others to love you? Are you ready to discover joy and living life as your true self?

Let's wrap up the book with the goal of starting your healing journey.

All it takes is ONE step, one change, to start your healing journey.

You don't need to attempt the herculean task of attempting to transform your life in one day. Start with *just one thing*... maybe start with what you eat; maybe go for a walk; visit your local park.

Last request. Healing and health and wellness is a lifelong pursuit, but we all have our limits, right? So, let's agree that once you begin your healing journey, you'll give the work at least six months to start taking effect, to start moving toward healing. And give yourself much grace as you move through the healing; you will face challenges — no doubt — but the life on the other side of that work is joyful, loving, freeing, and peaceful. And celebrate every little step of healing along the way — you deserve it!

As we wrap up this book, I want to point out one interesting thread that loops through all these healing modalities... and it has to do with the process of healing.

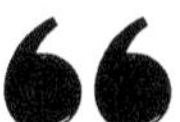

INSPIRING QUOTE

"Be kind to one another, tenderhearted, forgiving one another as God in Christ forgave you." — Ephesians 4:32

KEYS TO HEALING:

For every healing modality, here's what you have to do:

- **Intention**: If you want healing, you MUST be intentional about it. You must be clear that you want healing, are seeking healing: setting an intention that you will face whatever challenges you need to face in order to get healing.

- **Surrender**: In all things, you must surrender to the healing process. You have to find a way to release the ego into allowing the healing to take place. The surrendering you do in prayer or meditation is the same surrendering as done with psychedelics.
- **Integration**: With healing comes many realizations, changes, and revolutions. You must take the work you do in healing yourself and fully incorporate it into a new life, a new you — the TRUE you. Integration is all about taking these healing lessons and applying them to your entire life, including the people in your life.

Another piece of the healing process that needs to be discussed is forgiveness. The highest level of healing is when you can forgive the person (people) who have hurt you in the past. Note: You don't need to contact the person and forgive them; the forgiveness is for YOUR healing, not theirs.

AUTHOR INSIGHT

Surrender is so important to healing, and yet many people pause when hearing the word because it often relates to a sense of weakness or defeat. In this context, surrender means that we know we HAVE to HEAL and release all those unprocessed trauma responses... and it means an END of your pain and suffering. We surrender in these healing modalities, surrender our egos and our traumas, and we come away stronger, healthier, and truer (to our authentic selves).

I hear you. I have been there — on both sides of the equation. How can we possibly forgive someone who has caused us such deep pain, such hurt and damage to our psyche, our heart, our body? But you can — and must — because holding onto the pain and the hate and holding a grudge are all things that help block the healing.

HEALING HINT

Here's a beautiful meditation that is focused on forgiveness. In Ho'oponopono (a traditional Hawaiian practice of reconciliation and forgiveness), people use a repeated mantra: *I am sorry* (repentance); *please forgive me* (forgiveness); *thank you* (gratitude); *I love you* (love).

If you want healing, you have to forgive; and by forgive, it's best to define forgiveness as the intentional decision to let go of resentment and anger related to a specific event, a specific person.

WHY FORGIVENESS IS SO IMPORTANT:

1. It releases negative thoughts. It's about forgiving yourself for any involvement, including guilt and shame over the hurt. When you forgive, you move toward healing.
2. It helps get you out of victim mode. Forgiving is about releasing all that negative energy so that you can find true healing.
3. It's empowering for your self-esteem. When you choose to forgive someone who has hurt you, it puts all the power and emotional control back to you.
4. It's great for your health. If you're like me, when I am focused on something negative, it affects all other parts of my life; releasing that negativity allows us to focus on healing.
5. It can assist you in finding your true spiritual path. Forgiveness is a path toward peace; forgiveness can also be seen as an act of kindness.

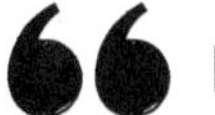

INSPIRING QUOTE

"Forgiveness is not always easy. At times, it feels more painful than the wound we suffered, to forgive the one that inflicted it. And yet, there is no peace without forgiveness." —Marianne Williamson

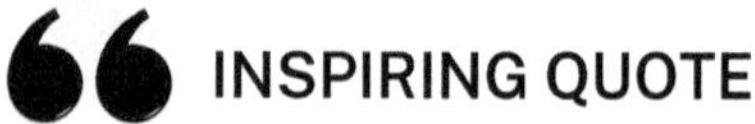

"The best six doctors anywhere — and no one can deny it — are sunshine, water, rest, air, exercise, and diet." —Wayne Fields

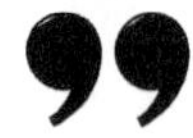

10 WHOLEISTIC TIPS FOR IMPROVING YOUR HEALTH, HEALING, AND LIVING YOUR BEST LIFE

1. **Heal Past Trauma.** So much of wellness is tied to past trauma — and the emotional responses trapped to that trauma — that we have to strive to heal first. Healing is the key that will help open all the other doors of a full and fulfilling life.
2. **Quit Smoking.** Everyone knows it's an unhealthy habit/addiction, and yet it can be so hard to finally quit. But know this, quitting smoking is beneficial to health at any age — and the sooner you quit, the sooner many others will be positively affected by no longer dealing with your secondhand smoke.
3. **Improve Nutrition.** Follow one of these mantras to better health: "We are what we eat" or "the body is a temple" or "food as medicine." The more you are healed and respect yourself, the more good foods and nutrition will be important to you.
4. **Follow Good Sleep Patterns.** We are not in a sleep crisis yet, but we're close, with 2 in 3 Americans reporting they are now sleeping either more or less than desired. Our bodies, souls, and minds need regular, high-quality sleep.
5. **Restrict Alcohol Consumption.** While drinking socially has almost always been acceptable, the science is revealing just how detrimental even small amounts of alcohol are to our health and well-being. As you heal, examine the role of alcohol in your life.

6. **Get Daily Exercise.** Exercise, of course, is one of the healing modalities, but here the emphasis is on making a conscious decision to physically move daily, which may include walking, biking, dancing, yoga, calisthenics, etc.
7. **Practice Spirituality.** Our egos can often get in the way of true healing, but when we begin to accept that there is some sort of higher being/power that created this world... and that we are ALL connected to each other, it helps reveal truths about the universe, consciousness, mysteries... the Divine.
8. **Focus on Mindfulness and Gratitude.** The easiest element of healing is taking time throughout your day to take mindfulness moments, a few minutes of peaceful thinking and gratitude. On those busier/crazier days, try to take more mindfulness moments.
9. **Perform Daily Breathwork Exercises.** These exercises are something you can do at your desk, on a break, at home... anywhere. You can do some short breathwork during the day and then when your workday is over, combine a little breathwork with a meditation for true peace and healing.
10. **Spend Time in Nature.** Even people living in the concrete jungle have access to parks, and you should consider taking time to sit on a park bench during a lunch break or perhaps before or after work. When sitting there in nature, you can also combine it with breathwork and meditation/prayer... even enjoy a healthy snack.

HEALING HINT

Magnesium is an essential mineral for our health – for a healthy body and brain. It helps with mood, sleep, and overall health. Every cell in our bodies uses magnesium – and yet most of us are critically deficient because of changes in agriculture and diet; it's believed that more than 70 percent of adults are deficient in magnesium.

BONUS TIP: Eliminate as much (if not ALL) negativity in your life — news, social media, people.

KEYS TO HEALING

Some key thoughts to remember about the healing process:

- It takes work, so be prepared to lean into your healing and commit the time and energy needed for true healing.
- Keep focused on gratitude, for the good things in your life and for all progress you make toward healing. A gratitude practice is essential.
- You need community to help heal, so keep working at finding your "tribe" — your people. You may also need to remove people from your life, so be prepared to grieve that loss.
- Sit through the pain of the release of the past trauma; avoiding it simply keeps it around.
- Keep moving forward and know that the healing process is not linear; expect some fits and starts and some struggles, but keep moving forward.
- When you're struggling with the progress — or the pain — seek help through a professional therapist, counselor, healer, or coach.

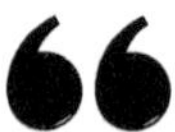

INSPIRING QUOTE

"... we have reached a point in our collective evolution where our health is being outpaced by lifestyles not aligned with how we are biologically designed to live. We are idle when our bodies want to move, we eat foods that are unrecognizable to our systems, and we expose ourselves to environmental factors that assault our cells." — Kelly Brogan, MD

FINAL THOUGHTS ABOUT HOLISTIC/WHOLEISTIC HEALING

The concepts outlined in this book are not original to me, but I have pulled these ideas from multiple sources and concepts, including the Medicine Wheel (or Sacred Hoop), a Native American approach to energy healing that looks more at stages of development, but is still a beautiful concept. (Learn more here: https://theshiftnetwork.com/blog/2019-04-05/seven-directions-medicine-wheel.)

Think of this book as your healing guide, a tool to assist you with uncovering, discovering, and celebrating your **true self**... *your authentic self.*

Depression, anxiety, OCD, addictions... these are just labels of outcomes from trauma. They are not a life sentence, but simply the result of trauma you experienced and could not process fully. Break free from these negative labels and find true healing through the tools in this book.

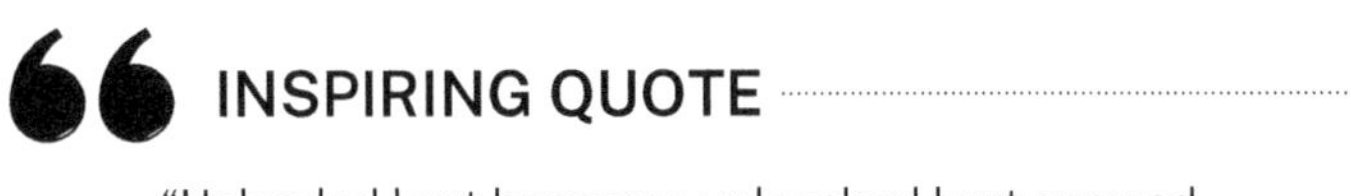

"Unhealed hurt becomes unleashed hurt spewed out on others." —Lysa Terkeurst

Finally, the coolest thing about wholeistic healing is that there is SO much overlap among the healing modalities... for example:

- Intentional psychedelic experience in nature;
- Breathwork combined with yoga or meditation;
- Somatic therapy or meditation or hiking in nature;
- Working in your garden, focused on better nutrition.

You now have all the tools you need to heal yourself — so please give yourself permission to go heal.

Stop managing symptoms! Heal!

You know you are on a healing path when...

- You begin to see hope for a better future;
- You are more emotional, as you get in touch with them;
- You start feeling more like yourself;
- You feel the positive changes taking hold;
- You see the real potential in fully healing;
- You begin to feel more love, peace, and joy.

PLEASE HEAL... first yourself; then help others.

As our wonderful American poet Maya Angelou wrote: "As soon as healing takes place, go out and heal somebody else."

Welcome to true healing and becoming the true (whole) you!

HEALING BOOKS AND DOCUMENTARIES

Books

If you are looking to take a deep dive into all the healing modalities, then this list of books should keep you busy for some time! Any and all of these books make an excellent addition to your healing library and to your greater understanding of health and healing.

About Psychedelic Healing

Triumph Over Trauma: Psychedelic Medicines are Helping People Heal Their Trauma, Change Their Lives, and Grow Their Spirituality, by Randall S. Hansen, Ph.D. 9798987252000. Written for those among us who are hurting, depressed, angry, and lost; for those seeking new treatments and true healing; for those searching for a higher purpose or a connection with the Divine; and for those simply curious about why the topic of psychedelics is seemingly everywhere. Highlight: 23 stories of transformation and healing through intentional use of psychedelics.

The Complete Guide to Microdosing Psilocybin Mushrooms | Guidebook & Journal: An All-Inclusive Beginners Guide to Microdosing Psilocybin Mushrooms & a Microdosing Journal, by Alan Alpert. 979-8845820686. An all-inclusive beginners guide to microdosing psilocybin mushrooms — along with a detailed microdosing journal for integration.

The Microdosing Guidebook: A Step-by-Step Manual to Improve Your Physical and Mental Health through Psychedelic Medicine, by C. J. Spotswood, PMHNP. 1646043103. Learn about the history, research, and helpful effects of microdosing psychedelic medicines like psilocybin, LSD, ecstasy, and more with this combination manual and workbook.

Psychedelics and Spirituality: The Sacred Use of LSD, Psilocybin, and MDMA for Human Transformation, edited by Thomas B. Roberts, Ph.D. 1644110229. Reveals how psychedelics can facilitate spiritual development and direct encounters with the sacred. With contributions by Albert Hofmann, Huston Smith, Stanislav Grof, Charles Tart, Alexander "Sasha" Shulgin, Brother David Steindl-Rast, and many others.

How to Change Your Mind: What the New Science of Psychedelics Teaches Us About Consciousness, Dying, Addiction, Depression, and Transcendence, by Michael Pollan. 1594204225. Presents a remarkable history of psychedelics and a compelling portrait of the new generation of scientists fascinated by the implications of these drugs.

Psychedelics For Everyone: A Beginners Guide to these Powerful Medicines for Anxiety, Depression, Addiction, PTSD, and Expanding Consciousness, by Matt Zemon. 979-8986267432. Provides readers with an inspiring foundation for understanding the profound transformational power of psychedelics, including medically-reviewed information from experts in the clinical use of psychedelics.

Cannabis Is Medicine: How Medical Cannabis and CBD Are Healing Everything from Anxiety to Chronic Pain, by Bonni Goldstein MD. 031650078X. Millions of people around the world are healing illnesses with cannabis. Nonetheless, many physicians remain reluctant to discuss cannabis medicine with their patients. This book is the comprehensive resource for people who have not found relief from conventional medicines.

The Doctor-Approved Cannabis Handbook: Reverse Disease, Treat Pain, and Enhance Your Wellness with Medical Marijuana and CBD, by Benjamin Caplan, MD. 1637742673. This is the science-backed, doctor-approved guide to cannabis for adults who are serious about improving their health. The medical benefits of cannabis have never been clearer. Dr. Caplan is a licensed, board-certified Family Physician who has overseen care of over 250,000 patients with guided cannabis care.

About Spiritual Healing

Altered Traits: Science Reveals How Meditation Changes Your Mind, Brain, and Body, by Daniel Goleman and Richard J. Davidson. 0399184392. In the last twenty years, meditation and mindfulness have gone from being kind of cool to becoming omnipresent tools for fixing everything from your weight to your relationship to your achievement level. This book showcases cutting-edge research that discusses what meditation can really do for us, as well as exactly how to get the most out of it.

The Art of Spiritual Healing, by Joel S. Goldsmith. 1939542685. A simple, straightforward explanation of what to many is a mysterious and complex subject. The book is presented in four parts: "The Principles," "The Role of Treatment," "The Practice," and "Without Words or Thoughts." Goldsmith believes that the world needs people who, through devotion to God, are so filled with the Spirit.

Healing the Emptiness: A Guide to Emotional and Spiritual Well-Being, by Yasmin Mogahed. B09XZH8DD4. In order to thrive, we need to know how to heal. This book is about finding strength in God and in our capacity to be both human and beautiful–both flawed and inspired. It is a journey to the understanding that we are flawed by design so that we can find strength and beauty in relying entirely on the Flawless.

Healing, Spiritual, and Esoteric Meditations: A Complete Guidebook to the Esoteric Spiritual Healing Path, by Georgios Mylonas. 197984190X. Healing, spiritual, and esoteric meditations to uplift your spirit, raise your consciousness, and guide you to experience the highest levels of illumination, enlightenment, and bliss! A complete guidebook to the esoteric spiritual healing path, featuring easy-to-follow, detailed and practical instructions, and guidelines for over 100 meditations, techniques, and visualizations.

Mindfulness Activities for Adults: 50 Simple Exercises to Relax, Stay Present, and Find Peace, by Matthew Rezac. 1638070539. This interactive book takes traditional mindfulness exercises and turns them into simple, engaging activities to bring any level of practitioner more calm and comfort.

Practicing Mindfulness: 75 Essential Meditations to Reduce Stress, Improve Mental Health, and Find Peace in the Everyday, by Matthew Sockolov. 1641521716. Even short meditations can turn a bad day around, ground us in the present moment, and help us approach life with gratitude and kindness. Find 75 essential exercises that offer practical guidance for anyone who wants to realize the benefits of mindful meditation.

Spiritual Activator: 5 Steps to Clearing, Unblocking, and Protecting Your Energy to Attract More Love, Joy, and Purpose, by Oliver Nino. 140196771X. Explains how energetic blocks lodge themselves in your system as negative beliefs, emotions, and sometimes even physical conditions. Traumas, ancestral roots, or environmental factors create feelings of fear, guilt, anger, betrayal, uselessness, hurt, and inadequacy that can flow through you like dangerous, free radicals.

Streams of Healing: Finding Your Way to Wholeness with Key Leaders in the Inner Healing Movement, compiled by Cathy Little and Melinda Wilson (with many contributors). B0BJ6LRXP2. Whether you are a counselor or minister looking for tools to help others, or you are new to your own healing journey, dive in and allow the current to take you farther and deeper into the healing power of Jesus.

About Somatic Healing

Somatic Therapy for Healing Trauma: Effective Tools to Strengthen the Mind-Body Connection, by Jordan Dann, LP. 1685393772. Trauma lives on in both the mind and the body, and focusing on the body-mind connection is a powerful tool for healing. This insightful workbook introduces you to somatic therapy, an approach that helps release emotional and physical stress that is trapped in the body, so you can process your trauma and begin to heal.

The Somatic Therapy Workbook: Stress-Relieving Exercises for Strengthening the Mind-Body Connection and Sparking Emotional and Physical Healing, by Livia Shapiro. 1646040953. The effects of a traumatic event are more than just mental. Trauma can manifest in the body as chronic pain, sluggishness, and depressed mood. Somatic psychology is an alternative therapy that analyzes this mind-body connection and helps you release pent-up tension and truly heal from past trauma.

Somawise: Get Out of Your Head, Get Into Your Body, by Dr. Luke Sniewski. 0989911179. The body lets us know through internal signals and cues when some aspect of our lifestyle is supporting or hindering the natural process of health. Start your journey back to yourself with the teachings and strategies provided in the book.

Therapeutic Yoga for Trauma Recovery: Applying the Principles of Polyvagal Theory for Self-Discovery, Embodied Healing, and Meaningful Change, by Arielle Schwartz, Ph.D. 1683735056. Trauma recovery is as much about healing the body as it is the mind, yet so often the focus of healing involves retelling the story of the past without addressing the physiological imbalances that trauma leaves in its wake. This book walks you through the sacred practice of yoga so you can release the burdens of trauma from your body and mind.

The Reiki Manual: A Training Guide for Reiki Students, Practitioners, and Masters, by Penelope Quest and Kathy Roberts. 158542904X. This comprehensive manual provides much-needed support for students and teachers who want to follow the best practices of Reiki. Includes coverage of Reiki levels 1, 2, and 3.

Sound Therapy & Energy Healing for Beginners: An Essential Guide, by Carmel Diviney. 979-8448982613. This essential guide is presented in an interesting and easy to follow style. You will learn how to harness and direct healing energy for self, family and friends, people at a distance and even your pets, trees, and plants.

Trauma Releasing Exercises (TRE): A Revolutionary New Method for Stress/Trauma Recovery, by David Berceli, PhD. 1419607545. The focus of the book is the ground-breaking, Trauma Releasing Exercises (TRE); these exercises elicit mild psychogenic tremors that release deep chronic tension in the body and assist the individual in the trauma healing process.

About Nature Healing

Forest Bathing: How Trees Can Help You Find Health and Happiness, by Dr. Qing Li. 052555985X. Notice how a tree sways in the wind. Run your hands over its bark. Take in its citrusy scent. As a society, we suffer from nature deficit disorder, but studies have shown that spending mindful, intentional time around trees–what the Japanese call shinrin-yoku, or forest bathing–can promote health and happiness.

Healing Trees: A Pocket Guide to Forest Bathing, by Ben Page. 1647224187. Intended as an easy approach to forest bathing, a concept that is now making its way into health and wellness practices. Part spiritual guide and part practitioner's handbook, this accessible, practical, positivity-rich book is designed to be taken on every walk to encourage mindfulness, contentedness, and presence in the moment.

Healing with Nature: Mindfulness and Somatic Practices to Heal from Trauma, by Rochelle Calvert, Ph.D. 1608687368. Shows how to relate to and connect with nature through the practice of mindfulness to calm and relax the nervous system, tune in to the somatic wisdom of the body to face lingering trauma and rewire it, and work with painful experiences to transform them in ways that heal the individual and contribute to healing the wider world.

Your Guide to Forest Bathing: Experience the Healing Power of Nature, by M. Amos Clifford. 1590035135. You'll discover a path that you can use to begin a practice of your own that includes specific activities. Whether you're in a forest or woodland, public park, or just your own backyard, this book will be your personal guide as you explore the natural world in a way you may have never thought possible.

About Breathwork Healing

Feel to Heal: Releasing Trauma Through Body Awareness and Breathwork Practice, by Giten Tonkov. 1797921630. Features successful body-based, trauma-release therapies to teach people how to break the trauma cycle, improve relationships, and achieve healthier, more fulfilling day-to-day lives. Periodically releasing trauma creates a "clean slate;" it also helps people to learn better how to deal with trauma when it occurs.

Holotropic Breathwork: A New Approach to Self-Exploration and Therapy, by Stanislav Grof and Christina Grof. 1438496443. Describes a groundbreaking form of self-exploration and psychotherapy: Holotropic Breathwork. Holotropic means "moving toward wholeness," from the Greek holos (whole) and trepein (moving in the direction of). The breathwork utilizes the remarkable healing and transformative potential of non-ordinary states of consciousness.

Just Breathe: Mastering Breathwork, by Dan Brule. 150116306X. gives you the tools to achieve benefits in a wide range of issues including: managing acute/chronic pain; helping with insomnia, weight loss, attention deficit, anxiety, depression, trauma, and grief; improving intuition, creativity, mindfulness, self-esteem, and leadership; and much more.

About Nutritional Healing

Encyclopedia of Healing Foods, by Michael T. Murray, ND, Joseph Pizzorno, ND, and Lara Pizzorno, LMT. 074348052X. The most comprehensive and practical guide available to the nutritional benefits and medicinal properties of virtually everything edible. Providing the best natural remedies for everyday aches and pains, as well as potent protection against serious diseases, The Encyclopedia of Healing Foods is a must-have daily health reference.

Healing Through Nature's Medicine: A Story of Hope, by Emanuela Visone, CHC, CLC. 9798668243754. "Through the concept of using nature's medicine, I want to open your mind to using this pure remedy so you don't look to medication as your first option. I am not a doctor, but I was my own living experiment. Slowly, I transformed and restored myself from chronic degenerative diseases. You too can heal your body naturally."

The Herbal Remedies & Natural Medicine Bible: 9 in 1. The Ultimate Guide to Build Your Apothecary Table. Use Healing Herbs & Medicinal Plants to Prepare Antibiotics, Tinctures, Teas, and Infusions, by Mary Paul. 9798377927754. A collection of powerful knowledge and wisdom in herbalism, botany, and holistic medicine. You get all the tools you need to finally get rid of common drugs and prepare your natural remedies. This book's step-by-step instructions will help you naturally explode your well-being.

Nutritional Healing Foods That Heal: Start Your Journey to a Mindful & Healthy Eating, by Dr. Louise Lily Wain. 9798635709955. Packed with practical strategies and heartfelt advice, this insightful book explores how you can heal your body and mind with the power of food. Diet is a long-forgotten method of healing that has been practiced for thousands of years—now, you can discover how to kickstart your health and well-being with all-natural fruits, herbs, spices, and more.

The Pegan Diet: 21 Practical Principles for Reclaiming Your Health in a Nutritionally Confusing World, by Dr. Mark Hyman. 1529329426. Using a food is medicine approach, Dr. Hyman explains how to take the best aspects of the paleo diet (good fats, limited refined carbs, limited sugar) and combine them with the vegan diet (lots and lots of fresh, healthy veggies) to create a delicious diet that is not only good for your brain and your body, but also good for the planet. Featuring 30 recipes, the book offers a balanced and easy-to-follow approach to eating that will help you get, and stay, fit, healthy, focused, and happy.

7 Steps to Get Off Sugar and Carbohydrates: Healthy Eating for Healthy Living with a Low-Carbohydrate, Anti-Inflammatory Diet, by Susan Neal, RN. 0997763663. Provides a day-by-day plan to wean your body off these addictive products and regain your health. These changes in your eating habits will start your lifestyle journey to the abundant life you deserve, not a life filled with disease and poor health. You will learn how to: eliminate brain fog, cure diseases, and lose weight.

General Healing

The Body Keeps the Score: Brain, Mind, and Body in the Healing of Trauma, by Bessel van der Kolk M.D. 0143127748. This book shows how trauma literally reshapes both body and brain, compromising sufferers' capacities for pleasure, engagement, self-control, and trust. The book explores innovative treatments — from neurofeedback and meditation to sports, drama, and yoga — that offer new paths to recovery by activating the brain's natural neuroplasticity.

Eight Weeks to Optimum Health: A Proven Program for Taking Full Advantage of Your Body's Natural Healing Power, by Andrew Weil, MD. An extremely practical week-by-week, step-by-step plan, covering diet, exercise, lifestyle, stress, and environment — all of the aspects of daily living that affect health and well-being.

In an Unspoken Voice: How the Body Releases Trauma and Restores Goodness, by Peter A. Levine PhD. 1556439431. This book draws on the author's broad experience as a clinician, a student of comparative brain research, a stress scientist, and a keen observer of the naturalistic animal world to explain the nature and transformation of trauma in the body, brain, and psyche.

The Myth of Normal: Trauma, Illness, and Healing in a Toxic Culture, by Gabor Maté MD. 0593083881. Western medicine often fails to treat the whole person, ignoring how today's culture stresses the body, burdens the immune system, and undermines emotional balance. Now this book attempts to untangle the common myths about what makes us sick, connects the dots between the maladies of individuals and the declining soundness of society.

The Pleasure Trap: Mastering the Hidden Force that Undermines Health and Happiness, by Douglas J. Lisle, PhD, and Alan Goldhamer, DC. 1570671974. This book boldly challenges conventional wisdom about sickness and unhappiness in today's contemporary culture, offers groundbreaking solutions for achieving change, and provides a fascinating new perspective on how modern life can turn so many smart, savvy people into the unwitting saboteurs of their own well-being.

The Transformation: The Path to Hope and Healing, by James Gordon, MD. 0062870726. In this compassionate and compelling book, the author invites us on a step-by-step, evidence-based journey to heal the psychological and biological damage that trauma brings and to become the people whom we are meant to be.

Transforming The Living Legacy of Trauma: A Workbook for Survivors and Therapists, by Janina Fisher. 1683733487. Traumatic experiences leave a "living legacy" of effects that often persist for years and decades after the events are over. Historically, it has always been assumed that retelling the story of what happened would resolve these effects; survivors need to understand their symptoms and reactions as normal responses to abnormal events.

What Happened to You? Conversations on Trauma, Resilience, and Healing, by Bruce D. Perry, MD, PhD, and Oprah Winfrey. Through deeply personal conversations, Oprah Winfrey and renowned brain and trauma expert Dr. Bruce Perry offer a groundbreaking and profound shift from asking "What's wrong with you?" to "What happened to you?"

Whole Body Healing: Create Your Own Path to Physical, Emotional, Energetic & Spiritual Wellness, by Emily A. Francis. 0738762180. Learn how to take an active role in your healing process and discover a wide range of treatment modalities to help you achieve physical, emotional, and spiritual wellness.

Documentaries

If you are more into sitting back and viewing, then these documentaries will make an excellent addition to your healing library and to your greater understanding of health and healing.

About Psychedelic Healing

Fantastic Fungi (2019). A consciousness-shifting documentary about the mycelium network that takes us on an immersive journey through time and scale into the magical earth beneath our feet, an underground network that can heal and save our planet.

Revealing the Mind: The Promise of Psychedelics (2019). A documentary that includes interviews with scientists and psychonauts who are now picking up where research left off 50 years ago when President Nixon made all psychedelics a Schedule 1 Drug, killing all the research being done on healing. Topics include LSD, psilocybin, DMT, and other psychedelics to heal — and reveal — the mind.

Hamilton's Pharmacopeia (2016-2019). From Hamilton Morris, the son of Errol Morris and a true science-geek, a multi-season docuseries that follows Hamilton's travels around the globe exploring the history, science, and social impact of psychoactive substances. Definitely a must-see.

How to Change Your Mind (2022). This series, based on the book by Michael Pollan by the same name, explores the history and use of psychedelics, including LSD, psilocybin, MDMA, and mescaline.

Psychedelica (2018-2019). A two-season docuseries that explores the history and use of psychedelic plants as a gateway to expanded consciousness and plant medicine's continued influence on humanity. Lots of great topics covered.

A Life of Its Own: The Truth About Medical Marijuana (2017). Award-winning journalist Helen Kapalos explores the subject of medical marijuana, uncovering life-changing treatments and cutting-edge research.

About Spiritual Healing

Conversations With God (2006). Chronicles the dramatic true journey of a struggling man turned homeless, who inadvertently becomes a spiritual messenger and bestselling author.

Happy (2011). Explores human happiness through interviews with people from all walks of life in 14 different countries, weaving in the newest findings of positive psychology.

Mantra: Sounds into Silence (2017). An uplifting documentary exploring the growing music and social phenomenon of chanting Mantras. It's a film about spirituality, not religion, where people reconnect with their true selves and with others.

Samsara (2011). Explores the marvels of the world and the richness of the human experience. Filmed across 25 countries over a five-year period and acclaimed for its mesmerizing visuals and music.

Unity (2015). A study in the duality of man. An examination of why humans can't get along with each other, the animals, or the environment, despite the advent of science, literature, technology, philosophy and religion.

About Nature Healing

The Hidden Life of Trees (2021). Renowned forester and writer Peter Wohlleben guides us through his most precious ideas and understanding of how trees work in this enlightening documentary.

How Forests Heal People (2017). A journey to discover the magical healing powers of nature. To find ways to reconnect people with nature through stories, films, and walks.

The Year the Earth Changed (2021). Narrated by David Attenborough, never-before-seen footage shows how our living in lockdown opened the door for nature to bounce back and thrive. Across the seas, skies, and lands, Earth found its rhythm when we came to a stop.

About Nutritional Healing

Cooked (2016). Acclaimed food writer Michael Pollan explores how cooking transforms food and shapes our world — through the lenses of the four natural elements — fire, water, air, and earth.

Food, Inc. (2008). Must-see. Narrated by Michael Pollan and Eric Schlosser, this documentary examines corporate/industrial farming, concluding that agribusiness produces food that is unhealthy in a way that is environmentally harmful and abusive of both animals and employees.

Rotten (2018). An investigative documentary series focusing on corruption in the global food supply chain, exposing the corruption, waste, and real dangers behind your everyday eating habits.

About General Healing

CrazyWise (2022). Crazy...or wise? The traditional wisdom of indigenous cultures often contradicts modern views about a mental health crisis. The film explores what can be learned from people around the world who have turned their psychological crisis into a positive transformative experience.

Heal (2017). Takes viewers on a scientific and spiritual journey where we discover that by changing one's perceptions, the human body can heal itself from any disease. Follows several individuals who used these techniques after being diagnosed with a fatal disease.

The Mind, Explained (2019). This docuseries is narrated by Emma Stone in Season 1 and Julianne Moore in Season 2, and examines themes such as what happens inside human brains when we dream or use psychedelic substances.

Take Your Pills (2018). In America today, where competition is ceaseless from school to the workforce and everyone wants a performance edge, Adderall and other prescription stimulants are the defining drugs of this generation.

ABOUT EMPOWERINGSITES.COM

Since 2007, EmpoweringSites.com has been a leader in publishing content that is designed to help people live better lives, starting first with wellness topics before expanding into healing.

The Empowering Sites Network is a content compendium with a mission to help you improve your life... all with free tools, expert advice, and links to the best resources.

EmpoweringSites.com is the corporate parent of several key websites, including:

- **HealMeWhole.com**
- **TriumphOverTraumaBook.com**
- **EmpoweringAdvice.com**
- **JenRanAdventures.com**
- **MyCollegeSuccessStory.com**
- **EmpoweringRetreat.com**

EmpoweringSites.com is also the publisher of two books focused on healing:

- ***Triumph Over Trauma***
- ***Heal!***

We are a small publishing company on a BIG mission of helping the world heal, live their best lives, and foster love and understanding.

Please join us on this mission by healing yourself and then sharing that healing with all the people you know.

To learn more, visit us at EmpoweringSites.com.

ACKNOWLEDGEMENTS

First and foremost, I have a big debt of gratitude for my storytellers; ordinary people who found healing and wanted to share that healing to help others, including **Angela, George, Daphne, TJ, Tristan, Megan, Louisa, Kat, Marissa,** and **Me'Shell**.

Second, I have to thank the coaches and healers who offered advice and tips, including **Kat Novotna, Marissa Kosolofski, Dr. Michael Hofrath, Bree Dellerson, Matt Simpson, Christopher Brown, Lizabeth Kashinsky,** and **Angela Lerro**.

Third, I have a special place in my heart for the wonderful people who offered early reviews of the book to help with the marketing of this important project, including **Jeff Bragg** and **Guy Borgford**.

Fourth, to my wonderful cousin, **Jennifer Smith**, who was working on her own book while I was working on mine; we spent a lot of time pumping each other up. Check out her book, *Warrior Fit Being Fit Isn't Just Physical: A Journey of Embracing Change, Empowering Your Whole Being, and Discovering the Warrior Within.*

Finally, I have to thank my wonderfully small team who have supported my healing work. First and foremost, the amazing, empathic, and lovely **Jenny Hansen**, a force in the veteran mental health and healing field. Second, the truly beautiful soul **Kelli Dickerson**, a critical thinker extraordinaire, and powerful supporter. Finally, the talented book designer and just wonderful human, **Michelle Fairbanks**.

NOTE TO THE READER

Thanks so much for taking the time to join me on this healing journey. I hope the words in this book will inspire you to seek healing — for yourself, a loved one, the world.

If the information here speaks to you — and you feel a need to share it — please consider posting a review on Amazon, Barnes & Noble, Goodreads... wherever books are reviewed. And if you do post a review, please share it on social media and tag me (see next page).

The more reviews, the more people can find true healing.

Finally, as I hope came across throughout the book, I wish you a beautiful and successful healing journey!

DR. RANDALL HANSEN'S CONTACT INFORMATION

Website: Randallshansen.com
LinkedIn: Linkedin.com/in/randallshansen
Facebook: Facebook.com/randallshansen/
Instagram: Instagram.com/empoweringpines/
X (Twitter): Twitter.com/rshansen/

www.ingramcontent.com/pod-product-compliance
Lightning Source LLC
Chambersburg PA
CBHW062114020426
42335CB00013B/960

* 9 7 9 8 9 8 7 2 5 2 0 2 4 *